The First Episode of Psychosis

T0346722

The First Episode of Psychosis

A Guide for Young People and Their Families

Revised and Updated Edition

Beth Broussard and Michael T. Compton

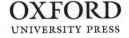

OXFORD
UNIVERSITY PRESS

OXFORD
UNIVERSITY PRESS

Oxford University Press is a department of the University of Oxford. It furthers
the University's objective of excellence in research, scholarship, and education
by publishing worldwide. Oxford is a registered trade mark of Oxford University
Press in the UK and certain other countries.

Published in the United States of America by Oxford University Press
198 Madison Avenue, New York, NY 10016, United States of America.

© Oxford University Press 2021

All rights reserved. No part of this publication may be reproduced, stored in
a retrieval system, or transmitted, in any form or by any means, without the
prior permission in writing of Oxford University Press, or as expressly permitted
by law, by license, or under terms agreed with the appropriate reproduction
rights organization. Inquiries concerning reproduction outside the scope of the
above should be sent to the Rights Department, Oxford University Press, at the
address above.

You must not circulate this work in any other form
and you must impose this same condition on any acquirer.

Library of Congress Cataloging-in-Publication Data
Names: Broussard, Beth, author. | Compton, Michael T., author.
Title: The first episode of psychosis : a guide for young people and their
families / Beth Broussard., Michael T. Compton
Description: Revised and Updated edition. | New York, NY : Oxford University Press,
[2021] | Includes bibliographical references and index.
Identifiers: LCCN 2020026338 (print) | LCCN 2020026339 (ebook) |
ISBN 9780190920685 (paperback) | ISBN 9780190920708 (epub) |
ISBN 9780197542514
Subjects: LCSH: Psychoses—Popular works.
Classification: LCC RC512 .C58 2021 (print) | LCC RC512 (ebook) |
DDC 616.89—dc23
LC record available at https://lccn.loc.gov/2020026338
LC ebook record available at https://lccn.loc.gov/2020026339

10.1093/med/9780190920685.001.0001

1 3 5 7 9 8 6 4 2

Printed by Marquis, Canada

Contents

Foreword   *vii*
Preface   *ix*
Acknowledgments   *xi*

PART I. ANSWERING SOME KEY QUESTIONS

1. What Is Psychosis?   3

2. What Are the Symptoms of Psychosis?   17

3. What Diagnoses Are Associated with Psychosis?   35

4. What Causes Primary Psychotic Disorders Like Schizophrenia?   49

PART II. CLARIFYING THE INITIAL EVALUATION AND
TREATMENT OF PSYCHOSIS

5. Finding the Best Care: Specialty Programs for Early Psychosis   59

6. The Initial Evaluation of Psychosis   69

7. Medicines Used to Treat Psychosis   83

8. Psychosocial Treatments for Early Psychosis   103

9. Follow-Up and Sticking with Treatment   119

PART III. HELPING YOU LOOK AHEAD TO THE
NEXT STEPS

10. Knowing Your Early Warning Signs and Preventing a Relapse   129

11. Staying Healthy   139

12. Embracing Recovery   149

13. Going Back to School and Work   155

14. Reducing Stress, Coping, and Communicating Effectively: Tips
    for Family Members and Young People with Psychosis   161

15. Understanding Mental Health First Aid for Psychosis   **173**

Glossary   *189*
Index   *213*

Foreword

The weeks and months during and following an initial episode of psychosis can be incredibly challenging, and also frightening, for young people, their families, and their broader social networks. During this period, access to reliable, up-to-date information is critical. This is exactly what this book provides: accurate and helpful information, resources, and support. The book educates readers about the symptoms of psychosis and how they are defined, the meaning of different diagnoses, and what the latest science tells us about underlying causes and effective treatments. Material covered includes the initial evaluation of psychosis, advances in the area of early intervention services, and information on evidence-based medications and psychosocial treatments. Importantly, chapters also provide practical advice on treatment engagement, relapse prevention, physical health and well-being, returning to school or work, and effective communication.

Since the first edition, much has changed in the treatment of first-episode psychosis. Specialized early intervention programs are now available in virtually every U.S. state, and in many parts of the world. These programs are team-based, recovery-focused, infused with shared decision-making, and centered around the young person's and family's own goals. The worksheets in this book—and the entire book itself—are designed to increase young people's and family members' knowledge and confidence, in turn strengthening communication with mental health professionals.

A fundamental message of this book is that treatment is effective and recovery is possible. I say that with confidence in part because I have been there: experiencing early psychosis, benefiting from specialized early intervention services, and now living a rich, and in many ways very "normal," life. Early in the course of psychosis it is of course easy to feel overwhelmed and hopeless; I encourage readers to always remain hopeful. While the challenges are real, thousands of young people in recovery, pursuing their goals, attest to the fact that challenges can be overcome. What can easily seem like a dead end in hindsight turns out to have been just a bend in the road. On that road, this book and the recovery-oriented supports it describes are a powerful resource on the journey to recovery.

Internationally, thousands of studies on psychosis are published every year. In this book, Beth Broussard and Michael Compton have distilled this science to what young people and families most need to know. Of course, mental health professionals will also share information tailored to individual situations, but the information contained in this book provides a comprehensive foundation regarding what we know about the causes, diagnosis, prognosis, and treatment of psychosis, and guidance on getting back on track. There are certainly still many things we don't fully understand about psychosis, but the field has made many important advances in the past decade and continues to move forward. This updated second edition reflects what we know and helps support the recovery process.

Nev Jones, PhD,
Assistant Professor, Morsani College of Medicine,
Department of Psychiatry and Behavioral Neurosciences,
University of South Florida,
Tampa, FL, USA

Preface

While the questions that open Chapter 1—often asked by young people experiencing psychosis and their families—might be the same as those from more than a decade ago when the first edition of this book was published, the answers have evolved. Treatment is getting better. Hope is more pertinent than ever before. Recovery and a full life are now achieved by many more people facing a first episode of psychosis. In this second edition, we share the latest information that we think will help you most effectively deal with this difficult situation. We have again aimed to provide readers with a complete guide explaining everything you need to know during this critical time of initial evaluation and treatment.

We often use the terms *first episode of psychosis*, *first-episode psychosis*, and *early psychosis*. They refer to the initial period of experiencing symptoms and the mental health evaluation and treatment for this episode of psychosis. Some individuals will go on to experience further episodes of psychosis, in which case the use of the term *first episode* is truly warranted. However, we do not mean to suggest that everyone who has a first episode of psychosis will necessarily go on to have future episodes. For some people, the symptoms clear up with treatment and they achieve long-term remission and recovery without later episodes.

We want to provide you with the information that you need to begin a path toward recovery or to go about helping your loved one embrace recovery. We invite you to read this book and gather from it whatever information is helpful to you. The book is divided into three parts, each one building on the next as you learn more about the first episode of psychosis. Important terms are shown in **bold** and definitions for each of these words are included in the glossary at the end of the book. We also invite you to visit a straightforward companion website for additional resources, including printable versions of the worksheets found in the book. Visit: www.oup.com/firstepisodepsychosis.

Hope and optimism for recovery are warranted, especially given the growing availability of specialty care. However, our optimism is balanced by a deep recognition of how serious the first episode of psychosis is. We strongly encourage young people and families to seek evaluation and treatment as soon as possible; to work together with experienced, specialized mental health professionals; and to stick with treatment. Through collaboration with experts in the treatment of psychosis, young people with psychosis and their families have the best chance to move beyond psychosis and toward recovery.

Beth Broussard, MPH, CHES,
Emory University School of Medicine,
Department of Psychiatry and Behavioral Sciences,
Atlanta, GA, USA
Michael T. Compton, MD, MPH,
New York State Psychiatric Institute and
Columbia University Vagelos College of Physicians and Surgeons,
Department of Psychiatry,
New York, NY, USA

Acknowledgments

We are delighted to be able to publish a thoroughly updated second edition that highlights the many advances of the past decade in early intervention services. Like the writing of the original text, this update and expansion has required substantial work, and we have benefited from the support and assistance of many. We would like to thank a number of dear colleagues who generously volunteered to review draft chapters for us, including Stephanie Langlois at DeKalb Community Service Board (Atlanta, GA); Robert Cotes at Emory University (Atlanta, GA); Leah Pope and Jason Tan de Bibiana at the Vera Institute of Justice (New York, NY); Tehya Boswell and Adria Zern at Columbia University (New York, NY); Nicole Havas at Lenox Hill Hospital and Northwell Health (New York, NY); and Iruma Bello, Leslie Marino, Hong Ngo, and Ilana Nossel at OnTrackNY (New York, NY). We are very fortunate to have such generous, hard-working, dedicated, and compassionate colleagues.

We also remain very appreciative of our former colleagues in the ACES Project (Atlanta Cohort on the Early Course of Schizophrenia) who helped us draft the original versions of chapters for the first edition, as well as the numerous international experts who reviewed those chapters. Their names are not repeated here, but much of their work undoubtedly carries over to this updated second edition. We continue to admire their research, clinical programs, and commitment to young people with first-episode psychosis and their families.

We also thank the many people important in both our professional and personal lives who have tolerated the long hours spent on compiling the original book, and the additional hours preparing this second edition. Their support and kindness remain essential to our success. At Oxford University Press, we thank Sarah Harrington for her ongoing encouragement, support, and assistance in guiding us through this project.

Finally, and most importantly, we acknowledge the young people who have experienced psychosis and their family members, who inspire us and continue to teach us that recovery is possible. We hope that our efforts will be helpful in their path toward recovery and embracing a meaningful, satisfying, and healthy life well lived.

B.B. and M.T.C.

PART I

ANSWERING SOME KEY QUESTIONS

1

What Is Psychosis?

What is happening? What are these voices? These odd and unusual ideas? What is causing it? What will the doctors do? Is this treatment necessary? Is this curable? Will it come back? How can our family cope? What should I do next?

These are some of the many questions that often go through the minds of young people experiencing psychosis and their family members. An episode of psychosis can be frightening. It can be confusing. It can even seem like life is changing forever. However, there is support for young people and their families. Know that treatment works, and recovery is possible. This book is meant to help readers through a very difficult time by providing much-needed information when taking the first steps toward recovery. Part I of this book, *Answering Some Key Questions*, explains some of the most important facts about psychosis. This chapter addresses the first question: What is psychosis?

In this chapter, we define what psychosis *is* and then dispel some myths by describing what psychosis is *not*. We then briefly describe what percentage of people develop psychosis and when it usually first begins. Next, we present the idea of a "psychosis continuum," which means that experiences of psychosis can differ in their level of seriousness. We then set the stage for later chapters by briefly introducing several other topics to come in the book, including causes of psychosis, treatments, and recovery.

What Psychosis Is

So what exactly does psychosis mean? **Psychosis** is a word used to describe a person's mental state when he or she has in some way become disconnected from reality. For example, a person might hear voices that are not really there (auditory hallucinations) or believe things that are not really true (delusions). It is a treatable mental illness that occurs due to a dysfunction in the brain. A **mental illness** affects a person's thoughts, feelings, and behaviors. You may be familiar with some other mental illnesses, such as depression, anxiety, and posttraumatic stress disorder. People with psychosis have difficulty separating false personal experiences from reality. They may have confusing speech patterns or behave in a bizarre or risky manner without realizing that they are doing anything unusual.

Similar to any other health condition, psychosis consists of a combination of different types of symptoms, which are described in detail in Chapter 2, "What Are the Symptoms of Psychosis?" Some of the many symptoms of psychosis may include hearing voices when there is really no one there, having unusual beliefs, feeling frightened or paranoid, being withdrawn, having confused thoughts or confusing speech patterns, or displaying odd behaviors.

A **psychotic episode** is a period of time during which someone has psychotic symptoms. These symptoms may make it difficult for the young person to carry out daily activities. A psychotic episode may last from days to weeks, or in some cases even months or years, depending on the person and whether treatment is received. In some cases, psychotic-like symptoms may last for only seconds or minutes but cause no problems or impairments, in which case they wouldn't be considered a psychotic episode.

People who have a **psychotic disorder** have a mental illness that interferes with their life. The various psychotic disorders and other illnesses that may cause psychosis are described in detail in Chapter 3, "What Diagnoses Are Associated with Psychosis?" Some people with a psychotic disorder have repeating episodes but are able to function normally between these episodes. Others may have repeating episodes without a full recovery between them. Yet others may have only one episode in their lifetime.

An episode of psychosis can seriously disrupt one's functioning. Both "positive symptoms," such as hallucinations and delusions (called "positive" because these symptoms are abnormal experiences *added on* to normal experiences), and "negative symptoms," such as decreased energy and motivation (called "negative" symptoms because they have *subtracted*, or removed, something from the person's experience), can interfere with school, work, and relationships. These and other types of symptoms are described in detail in Chapter 2.

Before a psychotic episode, family and friends may notice changes in emotions, behaviors, thinking, and beliefs about oneself and the world. They may see changes in mood, sleep habits, and participation in social activities. These changes, often called **prodromal symptoms**, are some of the early warning signs for a psychotic illness (see Chapters 2 and 10, "Knowing Your Early Warning Signs and Preventing a Relapse").

The experience of psychosis is different for each person. For some people, substance use, self-harm, or confusion may start or get worse with an episode of psychosis. Others may feel more tension or distrust. Family and friends should know that any unexpected or aggressive behavior is likely a reaction to hallucinations and/or delusions, which are very real for the person with psychosis. It is important to realize that unusual thoughts or behaviors are part of a treatable illness. Family and friends should understand that their loved one often does not have control over these thoughts and behaviors. Although the symptoms of psychosis may be frightening to the individual and his or her family, there are good treatments for these symptoms. Friends and family members should help the individual to receive the right mental health treatment.

First-episode psychosis is the period of time when a person first begins to experience psychosis. This book focuses on the first episode of psychosis because it is during this time that young people and their families need detailed information about the initial evaluation and treatment. The first few years during and after a first episode of psychosis is a critical period. That is, the early phase of psychosis is very important because it is during this time that long-term outcomes may be most improved by treatment. This is also a critical period because crucial psychological and social skills are developing, and mental health professionals want to minimize the interference to these skills that psychosis can cause. It is vital that individuals with psychosis and their families seek help in order to move toward recovery. The first episode of psychosis benefits most from specialized, thorough, and ongoing treatment that provides individuals with psychosis the best possible outcomes.

> It is vital that individuals with psychosis and their families seek help in order to move toward recovery. The first episode of psychosis benefits most from specialized, thorough, and ongoing treatment that provides individuals with psychosis the best possible outcomes.

What Psychosis Is NOT

Before learning more about psychosis, it is important to address some common myths and misconceptions about psychosis.

- **Psychosis is not multiple personality disorder.** In multiple personality disorder (a very rare psychiatric disorder that is now called dissociative identity disorder), a person unconsciously has two or more separate personalities. Each personality has its own thoughts, feelings, and behaviors. Although people with psychosis may hear voices or behave in response to delusions, they do not alternate between different personalities. So, psychosis is not "split personality" or multiple personality disorder.

- **Psychosis is not insanity.** The word *insanity* is a historical legal term that usually meant that one was too mentally ill to be held responsible for a crime (as in the phrase "not guilty by reason of insanity"). A very small percentage of individuals with psychosis and criminal charges fall into this legal classification. Usually, people with psychosis are not legally insane, nor do they usually commit crimes. Insanity is a word that is no longer used in the medical field.

- **People with psychosis are not "crazy."** People with psychosis should not be called crazy; instead, they are suffering from a treatable mental illness. Mental health professionals view the word *crazy* as an outdated and damaging word, like *insanity* or *lunacy*. Nowadays, mental health professionals encourage others not to use the word *crazy* because it leads to stigma and discrimination. People with a mental illness can still have friends and meaningful relationships, as well as go to school and have jobs. So, even though it is a commonly used word in society, referring to someone as "crazy" is harmful.

- **Psychosis is not psychopathy.** The word **psychotic** describes someone who is experiencing psychosis. Psychopathy is a personality disorder in which people lack empathy, have no regret for criminal or violent behaviors, and are socially manipulative. Although both mental illnesses contain the prefix *psycho*, they are completely different. Most people diagnosed with psychosis are not violent, and most people diagnosed with psychopathy (also called sociopathy or antisocial personality disorder) do not have hallucinations or delusions. So, psychosis does not equal psychopathy or criminal behavior.

- **Psychosis is not delirium.** People with delirium, or a state of confusion, may have trouble with memory and concentration. They may be disoriented, meaning that they do not know the date, where they are, or possibly even who they are (see Chapter 3). Although some people with psychosis have poor memory, they generally know who they are, where they are, and what the date is. So, psychosis is not the same as being delirious. Psychosis is also very different from dementia, which is a slowly developing state of confusion and memory loss that usually occurs in old age (see Chapter 3).

- **People with psychosis are not usually violent or a threat to others.** In fact, they are at greater risk for injuring themselves than injuring others. Family and friends should understand that people with psychosis are rarely violent. They are suffering from an illness and need the same caring attention as people with any other health condition.

- **Psychosis and disability do not always go hand in hand.** Recovery is possible. The experience of psychosis is different for every person who has it. Psychosis is more disabling for some people than for others because of individual differences in personality, social support, genes, and life experiences. The right treatment can help lessen or remove the distressing symptoms of the illness. Many people with psychosis can recover to participate in their communities.

Developing Psychosis

Psychosis affects both men and women across all cultures. When the symptoms of psychosis come together to form a syndrome that lasts for some time and causes impairment, it is often called a *psychotic episode*. That syndrome of psychosis, or the psychotic episode, can be classified into several different diagnoses, as described in Chapter 3, including psychotic disorders such as schizophrenia. Very few people (about 3%, or 3 in 100) will experience a psychotic episode in their lifetime. Although it can happen at any time in life, the onset or beginning of an episode of psychosis that is diagnosed as a psychotic disorder is usually in late adolescence or early adulthood. For men, the usual **age of onset** may be earlier than for women. That is, on average, men who develop a psychotic disorder experience their first psychotic symptoms up to three to five years before women do. For example, the symptoms of schizophrenia usually first become apparent in men between the ages of about 20 and 30, and in women between the ages of about 24 and 34. Schizophrenia is one of the most serious psychotic disorders, and about 1% of people will develop schizophrenia during the course of their lifetime.

The Psychosis Continuum

Everyone has some tendency to have psychotic-like experiences or even psychosis, just as everyone has the potential to become depressed or anxious. *Normal* experiences that are similar to psychosis, though much milder, do not interfere with an individual's regular functioning. *Abnormal* experiences of psychosis interfere with functioning and make it difficult for a person to live a regular life. The more an experience interferes with daily life, the more serious the condition.

Researchers who study psychosis use the phrase **psychosis continuum** to describe the different levels of experiences. This means that there is a range of **severity** or seriousness across the different types of experiences of psychosis. The different types of experiences range from normal experiences that are similar to psychosis and that cause little or no distress, to the full syndrome of psychosis that causes much distress or many difficulties in life. Although normal psychotic-like experiences are fairly common, psychotic disorders that cause the full syndrome of psychosis are quite rare. Figure 1.1 illustrates how the different types of experiences of psychosis relate to one another. The following five paragraphs relate to the five parts of Figure 1.1.

First, some normal human experiences that do not affect regular functioning are similar to psychosis. They cause no distress and do not interfere with life. We have all had the occasional experience of wondering if someone might be talking about us (which is a normal curiosity) or thinking that we hear the phone ring while taking a shower (which is a normal experience of attention being drawn to sounds that may be heard over noise). Some people occasionally may have minor psychotic-like symptoms, such as hearing a voice or suspecting that someone is following them. These brief, infrequent symptoms do not disrupt functioning. About one-fourth (25%, or 25 out of 100) of people in the general population will experience these types of symptoms at some point in their lifetime. These are brief experiences that usually go away, and not the full syndrome of psychosis. Psychosis is an exaggeration of these experiences—to the point that they become troubling and interfere with life—caused by a dysfunction in the brain.

Second, certain experiences can cause a psychotic episode, such as major stress, drug use, and even some medical problems. Some examples of psychosis caused by stressors include **stress-induced psychosis, drug-induced psychosis**, and **psychosis related to a medical problem**. People who experience a great deal of physical stress from lack of sleep, hunger, torture, or severe psychological stress, may experience stress-induced psychosis. Drug-induced psychosis may happen when a person is using drugs like cocaine, LSD, marijuana, methamphetamine, PCP, or synthetic cannabinoids. People with certain physical illnesses, such as meningitis, certain types of seizures, or a brain tumor, may experience psychosis related to a medical problem (see Chapter 3). In all of these cases, the symptoms of psychosis often, but not always, go away after removing the stressor, drug, or medical problem. Some people do not fully recover from an episode of psychosis if the stressor or cause of psychosis is too intense or lasts for too long, or if they are at genetic risk for a psychotic illness.

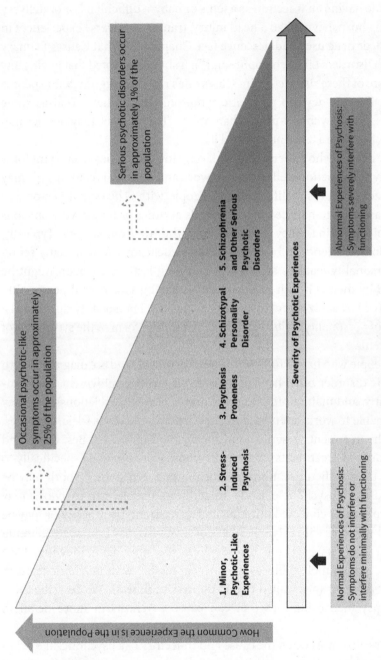

Figure 1.1 The Psychosis Continuum. Shown here is the range of severity among the different types of psychotic-like and full psychotic experiences. These experiences range from experiences that produce no or minimal levels of distress (left side) to those that cause a lot of distress (right side).

Third, some people are particularly at risk for psychosis due to their genes or due to exposure to factors that may have occurred in early life. Such factors may include having an infection as a fetus or baby, a difficult labor or delivery when being born, having had a head injury, trauma or adverse experiences in childhood, or drug use in adolescence (see Chapter 4, "What Causes Primary Psychotic Disorders Like Schizophrenia?"). It should be noted that having any one or more of these risk factors increases one's risk only slightly. Some people are more likely to develop psychotic symptoms than others. That is, some people are more **psychosis-prone** than others. They may or may not develop psychosis, but have a tendency toward it.

Fourth, people who experience mild, ongoing difficulties from symptoms but usually still function well enough to work and maintain relationships may have **schizotypal personality features**. People with schizotypal personality features can seem to have fewer social skills at times or may have suspicious or paranoid thinking. They also tend to withdraw from society. Typically, they do not experience full hallucinations or delusions. When many schizotypal personality features are present and long-lasting, a person might be diagnosed by mental health professionals as having **schizotypal personality disorder** (or just **schizotypal disorder**). Schizotypal personality disorder is a stable set of personality traits that appear as a milder form of the symptoms of schizophrenia.

Fifth, people who have a full syndrome of psychosis and are diagnosed with a psychotic disorder often have more difficulty with employment, living independently, and maintaining personal and professional relationships. They may be unable to work, attend school, or participate in some social activities. Some of the treatments described in Chapters 5, "Finding the Best Care," and 8, "Psychosocial Treatments for Early Psychosis," are designed specifically to help with these difficulties. Either hallucinations, delusions, or both may be present during a psychotic episode. In addition, people with psychosis may experience slow or confused thinking and speech, and their behavior may be odd or risky. People with this experience of psychosis may have schizophrenia or another "primary psychotic disorder." On the other hand, they may have a different type of mental illness, such as depression with psychotic features or bipolar disorder (also called manic-depressive illness). We describe these different psychiatric illnesses that can cause psychosis in more detail in Chapter 3.

There are also cases when the cause and trajectory of a psychotic-like experience are not clear. For example, some people have reported abilities related to their spirituality or religion, such as seeing or hearing things that other people cannot. These experiences usually do not interfere with an individual's functioning, and one's specific religion or culture considers them to be normal or special experiences. This book focuses on the types of experiences of psychosis that are abnormal or distressing.

Schizophrenia and Other Primary Psychotic Disorders

When someone has a headache, he or she may not know what is causing the headache. Is the headache from stress? Does the person have a cold or the flu? Or is the headache related to something more serious, like high blood pressure, or even a brain tumor? If the headache worsens or does not go away, it is a good idea to visit the doctor for medical evaluation and treatment. In the same way, psychosis can happen in several different illnesses, mostly in mental illnesses. For example, people with severe depression, with bipolar disorder, or with schizophrenia can have an episode of psychosis. There are many different types of psychotic disorders, and they are diagnosed based on the types of symptoms and how long those symptoms last.

For example, schizophrenia is a type of psychotic disorder in which at least two of the following occur for at least one month, but often much longer: hallucinations, delusions, disorganized speech, disorganized behavior, or "negative symptoms" (these symptoms are described in Chapter 2). Young people, in the age range of about 16 to 30, with a first episode of psychosis may or may not go on to develop schizophrenia. Nevertheless, mental health professionals always recommend a thorough evaluation (see Chapter 6, "The Initial Evaluation of Psychosis"), treatment (see Chapters 7, "Medicines Used to Treat Psychosis," and 8), and follow-up (see Chapter 9, "Follow-Up and Sticking with Treatment").

Schizophrenia is only one type of psychotic disorder, as described in Chapter 3. Others include brief psychotic disorder, schizophreniform disorder, schizoaffective disorder, and delusional disorder. These disorders differ from schizophrenia by the types of symptoms present and the length of time those symptoms last.

Psychotic disorders have a unique set of symptoms that make them different from other mental illnesses, placing them in their own class of disorders. All mental illnesses are defined by a specific group or set of symptoms. For example, people with obsessive-compulsive disorder do not have hallucinations, but people with psychosis often do. In other words, the symptoms of obsessive-compulsive disorder, depression, social anxiety disorder, autistic disorder, or a number of other mental illnesses differ from the symptoms of psychosis.

Possible Causes of Psychosis

Although Chapter 4 goes into detail about the causes of psychosis, it is important to begin to understand the causes here. Psychosis researchers believe there are two main models for the causes of the illness. These two models are not competing; they go hand in hand. One involves the developing brain (**neurodevelopmental model**), and the other is about the relationship between genes and stress (**diathesis–stress model**).

Psychosis is a medical condition of the brain, but scientists have not figured out exactly what is happening in the brain to cause this illness. Some think that it is a result of minor injuries to the brain during its growth and development or biological mishaps during brain development. They call this idea the *neurodevelopmental model*. Problems with brain development can happen for several reasons, as described further in Chapter 4.

Adolescence is a time when the brain goes through major changes. The minor brain injuries that may have happened during fetal brain development may become more apparent in adolescence when the brain develops further. These injuries can start to affect a person's thinking, feelings, and behavior. That is, some doctors and researchers think that psychosis happens as an individual is maturing in adolescence because he or she was born with minor brain development problems. This view explains why psychotic illnesses rarely occur in young children. Additionally, it can explain why first-episode psychosis is most common in late adolescence and young adulthood.

The other main explanation for why psychosis happens involves the relationship between genes and risk factors in early life. In this diathesis–stress model, it is thought that some people are born with genes that put them at greater risk for having psychosis. However, according to this model, it is thought that genes alone may not be enough to start a psychotic episode; there must also be a stressor to trigger an episode, such as a stressful life event or drug use. The combination of certain genes and a stressor can cause psychosis. Again, Chapter 4 provides much more detail on the causes of psychotic disorders like schizophrenia.

Taking Action: Treatment and Recovery

There are three phases of psychosis. The first is the **prodromal phase**, the time before a psychotic episode begins, when subtle symptoms may first appear. The prodromal phase may last from several weeks to several years. It is often not recognized as the early stages of a mental illness. The **acute phase** is the time during the psychotic episode when symptoms are most disrup-tive. The acute phase usually lasts until treatment is sought and symptoms are first evaluated and treated. The third is the **recovery phase**, the time after the episode when symptoms of psychosis lessen or sometimes go away com-pletely with treatment. The recovery phase is often considered to be the first 6 to 18 months of treatment.

People who get into treatment earlier often do better. In many places, spe-cialty treatment programs now exist that specifically focus on first-episode psychosis. They often provide treatments designed to help young people with psychosis get back on track in terms of school and work goals. The best help for someone with psychosis is to be active about seeking treatment and following through completely with treatment. To be active about seeking treatment means doing several things. It means going to see a mental health professional as soon as any disturbing symptoms appear. It also means learning about psy-chosis by talking to others or reading books. There are many resources in the community, as well as on the internet, to help understand this experience. When going to the mental health professional, do not hesitate to ask questions or express concerns. Psychosis is a treatable mental illness.

> People who get into treatment earlier often do better. In many places, specialty treat-ment programs now exist that specifically focus on first-episode psychosis. They often provide treatments designed to help young people with psychosis get back on track in terms of school and work goals.

An episode of psychosis can be a frightening and stressful experience for both the person with psychosis and their loved ones. Untreated psychosis can disrupt the life of both the individual and their family and friends. It is per-fectly understandable that both the person and their family members would feel scared, disappointed, or upset when dealing with the new onset of psy-chotic symptoms. Psychosis, though often frightening and confusing, should be treated promptly when at all possible, like any other illness.

For many individuals with first-episode psychosis, their "positive" psy-chotic symptoms (such as hallucinations or delusions) will clear up par-tially or completely within weeks of starting treatment. Treatment includes both medicine (see Chapter 7) and psychosocial treatments (see Chapter 8). Hospitalization is sometimes needed, as described in Chapter 6. Nowadays, even though psychiatric inpatient units might be "locked" (such that indi-viduals receiving treatment can't simply walk out), treatment strives to be compassionate, of high quality, and effective, with the stay being as short as possible, and the individual and family having a voice in decisions. In many settings, a typical hospital stay for the evaluation and treatment of an episode of psychosis might be several days or up to a couple of weeks, with 7 to 10 days often being about the average. Then, outpatient treatment becomes very important. Following through with treatment is crucial for recovery. Recovery, which is much broader than just eliminating symptoms, is described in detail in Chapter 12.

Putting It All Together

Psychosis is a treatable disorder of the brain that disrupts an individual's ability to understand the difference between personal experiences and reality (for example, hearing voices or having unusual beliefs). Many of society's ideas about psychosis are not true, such as the notion that people with psychosis have multiple personality disorder, are insane, are dangerous, or cannot recover. Everyone has the potential to experience some psychotic-like experiences or even psychosis. The continuum of psychosis ranges from normal, everyday experiences that interfere very little in people's lives to more serious experiences that greatly interfere with everyday life. The different psychotic disorders vary in the types and duration of symptoms associated with them. We explain these symptoms and diagnoses in Chapters 2 and 3.

While the exact cause of psychosis is not yet known, there are two main hypotheses. One is the neurodevelopmental hypothesis, which means that psychosis is a result of minor injuries to the brain during its growth and development or biological mishaps during brain development. The second is the diathesis–stress model, which means that psychosis is a result of the relationship between genes and factors in early life.

> Even though researchers are still trying to figure out the exact causes of psychosis, effective treatments are available. For most people with psychosis, many symptoms clear up with treatment, and they can move forward with their life goals through recovery.

Even though researchers are still trying to figure out the exact causes of psychosis, effective treatments are available. For most people with psychosis, many symptoms clear up with treatment, and they can move forward with their life goals through recovery. It is important to actively seek treatment and stick with it. This will help to increase chances of recovery and reduce relapse and rehospitalization.

Key Chapter Points

- Psychosis is a treatable mental illness. A mental illness affects a person's thoughts, feelings, and behaviors. For many people with first-episode psychosis, symptoms begin to clear up partially or completely within weeks of starting treatment.
- Although the symptoms of psychosis may be frightening to the individual and his or her family, there are some good treatments for these symptoms. Friends and family members should help the individual receive the right mental health treatment.
- First-episode psychosis is the period of time when a person first begins to experience psychosis. It is during this time that young people with psychosis and their families need detailed information about the initial evaluation and treatment.
- Young people, in the age range of about 16 to 30, with a first episode of psychosis may or may not go on to develop schizophrenia. Nevertheless, mental health professionals always recommend a thorough evaluation, as well as treatment with both medicine and psychosocial treatments.
- People who get into treatment earlier often do better. In many places, specialty treatment programs now exist that specifically focus on first-episode psychosis. They often provide treatments designed to help young people with psychosis get back on track in terms of school and work goals.

2

What Are the Symptoms of Psychosis?

Before learning about the symptoms of psychosis, it is important to understand what healthcare providers mean by the words *symptoms*, *signs*, *syndromes*, and *diagnosis*.

Nearly any illness, whether it affects the body or the brain, causes **symptoms**. A symptom is an obvious change from one's normal health that happens when an illness or disease occurs. For example, symptoms of a heart attack may include chest pain, pressure in the chest, pain running down the left arm, problems breathing, nausea, and sweating. Symptoms of the flu may include fever, chills, cough, sore throat, and nausea. Symptoms often are the reason you go to a doctor or other healthcare provider. The doctor then examines the person to look for **signs**. Signs are like symptoms, but a doctor sees them through an interview, exam, or test. In contrast, symptoms are experienced by the individual, who may not even know that he or she has signs of an illness. For example, during a routine checkup, the doctor may discover that a person has high blood pressure or high cholesterol. These signs, even if the person was not aware that they had existed, could mean that one has heart disease or is at risk for a heart attack. So, *symptoms* are experienced by the person with the illness, and *signs* are observed or detected by others.

Most medical diseases and mental illnesses cause both symptoms that one experiences and signs that doctors and other healthcare providers observe. A combination of both symptoms and signs is a **syndrome**. A heart attack is an example of a medical syndrome. Another example, diabetes, has symptoms such as being thirsty and frequent urination, and signs such as high levels of sugar in the blood. There also are many types of mental illness syndromes, such as depression, panic attacks, psychosis, and dementia. This book focuses on the syndrome of psychosis and the first time it appears. This usually happens between the ages of 16 and 30 years.

The distinction between *signs* and *symptoms* is sometimes important. For example, some features of psychosis might not be apparent to the person experiencing them at all. Many people who have some of the features described below, like "flat affect," "slow or empty thinking," "disorganization," and "impaired insight," might be completely unaware of them. Only others can see it and understand that it is happening. In such cases *symptom* is a misnomer (as the person isn't experiencing it as a problem), and *sign* is the more correct medical term. However, throughout the rest of this chapter and the chapters that follow, we use the term "symptom" to include both symptoms and signs. Doing so is easier than always classifying a feature of psychosis as either a symptom or a sign. The key is to learn the various features of psychosis, without always having to call some of them "signs" rather than just "symptoms."

The word **diagnosis** (or the plural, **diagnoses**) refers to the specific medical term given to an illness or syndrome by healthcare providers. Examples of medical diagnoses include "diabetes mellitus" (diabetes) and "acute myocardial infarction" (heart attack). Diagnoses of mental illnesses include "bipolar disorder" and "major depressive disorder." As discussed in Chapter 3 ("What Diagnoses Are Associated with Psychosis?"), the diagnoses of "brief psychotic disorder," "schizophreniform disorder," "schizophrenia," "schizoaffective disorder," and "delusional disorder" form a category of illnesses called *primary psychotic disorders*, because they all cause psychosis.

Like many other mental illnesses, early psychosis is a syndrome that causes many different symptoms. Different people experiencing psychosis have different types of symptoms, and one person's symptoms may change during his or her illness. In this chapter, you will learn about nine groups of symptoms that may happen during early psychosis (Table 2.1). The first three, positive symptoms, negative symptoms, and disorganized symptoms, are thought by some to be the three main groups of symptoms in primary psychotic disorders like schizophrenia. However, there are several other groups of symptoms that also may lead to difficulties, including impaired insight, cognitive dysfunction, hostile/aggressive symptoms, catatonic and movement symptoms, mood symptoms and anxiety, and suicidal thoughts. All of these are described in this chapter.

We also discuss prodromal symptoms at the end of this chapter. Prodromal symptoms actually happen *before* psychosis begins. If you or someone you know has had an episode of psychosis, you may recall some of the milder symptoms that appeared before the psychotic symptoms began. These are important to learn about even though they happened in the past because a period of prodromal symptoms often occurs before a future relapse or another episode of psychosis.

Table 2.1 Nine Types of Symptoms of Early Psychosis

Type	Description
Positive Symptoms	Things that young people should not normally do or think. In other words, these symptoms are abnormal experiences added on (which is why they are called "positive") to normal psychological experience.
Negative Symptoms	Things that people should normally do or think but are now missing. In other words, these symptoms have subtracted, or removed, something from their experience (which is why they are called "negative symptoms").
Disorganization	Sometimes in psychosis the normal flow of thinking and speaking can become out of order, confusing, or jumbled. Individuals can also experience difficulties with the ability to think clearly.
Impaired Insight	Often referred to as an unawareness of illness. People experiencing psychosis may not realize that the thoughts and behaviors they are having are a change from their previous self and that their behavior is different from that of others.
Cognitive Dysfunction	Causes difficulties with concentration, learning, memory, and planning. Individuals may also have some difficulties with specific cognitive abilities, like the ability to understand, process, and recall information.
Hostile/Aggressive Symptoms	Although rare, hostility and aggression are usually driven by specific delusions or paranoia and individuals may act out of fear. Individuals may argue more than normal, destroy property, or make threats toward others.
Catatonic/Movement Symptoms	A severe change from normal body movements that happens without a clear reason. Individuals may lose the ability to move, appearing frozen, stiff, and motionless.
Mood Symptoms and Anxiety	People with psychosis may experience depression, or periods in which they feel abnormally high or energetic, known as mania. Being anxious or nervous, sometimes due to delusional thoughts, is also common. Individuals may be tense or jittery, worry that something bad is going to happen, or appear generally uneasy.
Suicidal Thoughts	Thoughts about dying, including wishing to be dead, as well as thinking about or planning to commit suicide. These may be driven by symptoms or insight into how the person has changed. As young people experiencing psychosis for the first time are at an increased risk of suicide, any expression of suicidal thoughts should be taken very seriously.

Positive Symptoms

The most outwardly obvious symptoms of psychosis are **positive symptoms**. The use of the word "positive" is often confusing: It does not mean that these symptoms are enjoyable or helpful. They are things that young people should not normally do or think. In other words, these symptoms are abnormal experiences *added on* (which is why they are called "positive") to normal psychological experience. Positive symptoms include hallucinations, delusions, suspiciousness/paranoia, and ideas of reference. Each of these is discussed in the pages that follow.

Hallucinations

A **hallucination** is a false experience of one of the five senses (hearing, seeing, feeling, smelling, and tasting). Even though hallucinations may happen in any of the five senses, **auditory hallucinations** are the most common. Auditory hallucinations occur when someone hears voices, even though no one is speaking. These hallucinations may be voices calling one's name, commenting on one's actions, making harsh comments, or giving commands. Individuals with psychosis may react to the voices they are hearing—such as by talking to oneself, whispering to oneself, or looking around as if someone else is talking. The voices are not made up or imagined; the person who hears them is actually hearing the voice because of an abnormality in the brain. It is important to realize that the experience is very real to the person experiencing hallucinations.

Delusions

A **delusion** is a false belief that lasts for a long time. There are several different types of delusions:

- A **paranoid delusion** is the false belief that one is being plotted against or followed. For example, a person may believe that the police have planted a camera in the walls and his or her family is part of a government plot.
- A **grandiose delusion** is the false belief that one has high social status, is famous, has large amounts of money, or has special powers.
- A **religious delusion** is the false belief that one has religious importance, such as being a biblical figure.

- A **somatic delusion** is the false belief that something is wrong with one's body. For example, a person may believe that there is a parasite in his or her skin or that a cancer or tumor is growing in his or her body.
- A **delusion of control** is the false belief that some other person or an outside force controls one's thoughts, feelings, or actions. For example, a person may be convinced that someone else is putting thoughts into his or her mind through a hex, a curse, or some other means.

Mental health professionals refer to delusions as *bizarre* when they are clearly impossible. The belief that a remote control is influencing one's sense of smell is an example of a bizarre delusion. Other delusions are "non-bizarre" if they could happen but are clearly false for this particular person (such as being followed by multiple different black vehicles, your food being poisoned, or a drug dealer being out to get you). It is important to note that delusions are not just ideas or passing thoughts; rather, they are firmly held beliefs. Even though some psychosocial interventions, like cognitive-behavioral therapy (see Chapter 8, "Psychosocial Treatment for Early Psychosis"), may gently address the false nature of delusions, it is usually not helpful to try to "talk someone out of their delusions" or try to prove the person wrong. People with one or more delusions believe these ideas just like they believe anything else about themselves. It is their reality.

Suspiciousness/Paranoia

People with psychosis may experience **suspiciousness** and cannot trust others. They may have an unexplained feeling that those around them are trying to cause problems in their life. Sometimes this suspiciousness may be so severe that it is a paranoid delusion as described earlier. Other suspiciousness may be milder and result in people isolating themselves from others because they do not trust them. People with paranoia may not ask for help because they believe that others are trying to harm them rather than help them.

Ideas of Reference

Ideas of reference occur when people believe that others are talking about them or that things are referring especially to them when they really are not. For example, someone might believe that the television or radio newscasters are talking about them or are trying to send coded messages. This might prompt the person to remove or even destroy the television or radio because of these troubling ideas.

More than one positive symptom may occur at a time. The presence of one or more positive symptoms means that one has psychosis. For example, a person might hear a male voice repeatedly saying that things are not safe outside (auditory hallucinations). That same person might believe that the voice is coming from the apartment downstairs—a neighbor trying to keep them from feeling safe and from going to the clinic (a delusion). Experiencing either or both of those symptoms means that the person has psychosis and could have a primary psychotic disorder, which will be covered in Chapter 3.

Negative Symptoms

Another group of symptoms related to psychosis are the **negative symptoms**. Negative symptoms are things that people should normally do or think but are now missing. In other words, these symptoms have *subtracted*, or removed, something from their experience (which is why they are called "negative symptoms"). Some negative symptoms include anhedonia; apathy; blunted affect or flat affect; emotional withdrawal; low drive, energy, or motivation; poor attention to grooming and hygiene; slow or empty thinking and speech; slow movements; and social isolation:

- **Anhedonia:** Anhedonia is a loss of interest or pleasure. People experiencing this symptom may not be able to find pleasure in things that they used to enjoy. They also may find that they are unable to fully enjoy fun and pleasant things like going to the movies, enjoying a tasty meal, or taking part in hobbies.
- **Apathy:** People with apathy tend not to care as deeply about what happens in their life. This may include not being upset about negative life events such as losing a job or failing in school.
- **Blunted affect:** People with blunted affect show less outward emotion than normal. This is observed as decreased facial expression, less use of body language, and a dull tone of voice. A **flat affect** is a more serious loss of outward emotion, worse than blunted affect. People with a flat affect have an almost complete absence of facial expressions and body language, resulting in a very dull appearance and tone of voice.
- **Emotional withdrawal:** People with emotional withdrawal lack emotional closeness to others. They do not feel like they belong or connect with others, even when spending time with other people.

- **Low drive, energy, or motivation:** Young people experiencing this symptom may have lost the desire to finish school, to be in a relationship, to get a job, or to participate in social activities.
- **Poor attention to grooming and hygiene:** Poor attention to grooming and hygiene can include not bathing, not brushing one's teeth, wearing dirty clothes, or not combing one's hair. This neglect can happen for many reasons; for example, it may be the result of other negative symptoms, like apathy and low motivation.
- **Slow or empty thinking and speech:** People experiencing this symptom may seem like they are unable to keep up with the conversation. There may also be a long period between asking a question and their response to it. It may seem like they have very few thoughts.
- **Slow movements:** Individuals with slow movements as a negative symptom may walk, move, and talk more slowly than normal.
- **Social isolation:** People experiencing social isolation may become unconcerned with relationships that had been close and important to them before. They usually have difficulty forming new relationships. They may instead spend most of their time alone.

While these negative symptoms are less obvious than positive symptoms, they can make it very hard to attend school, keep a job, and have relationships. People should not mistake negative symptoms for laziness or an attitude problem. This wrongly blames the individual for serious symptoms that are not under his or her control. Many of the negative symptoms are very similar to symptoms of depression. However, in the case of psychotic disorders, the emotional tone underpinning negative symptoms is anhedonia (loss of interest) and apathy (not caring as deeply), rather than sadness and depression.

Although positive symptoms tend to alternate between better and worse over time, negative symptoms are often longer-lasting. Unfortunately, the medicines currently available are less effective at treating negative symptoms than positive symptoms (see Chapter 7, "Medicines Used to Treat Psychosis").

Disorganization

Sometimes in psychosis, there are signs of **disorganization** of thoughts and speech. The normal flow of thinking and speaking can become out of order, confusing, or jumbled. Two examples of disorganization of thoughts are tangentiality and loosening of associations:

- **Tangentiality:** Tangentiality happens when one idea connects to the next, but the thoughts become confusing because they go off on a tangent and end on a different subject. Tangentiality might sound like this: "I'm hungry. I need to go to the store to get a loaf of bread because bread is the staff of life. The staff members at my college seem too busy. They need more help. They need to hire more people to help them. Especially because the unemployment rates are high. It's not good to be unemployed. Congress really needs to do something about it ..." Here, the person starts talking about one topic but veers off on an unrelated tangent and never gets back to the original topic.
- **Loosening of associations:** Unlike tangentiality, loosening of associations (also called **derailment**) is when one idea does not match the next at all. The ideas do not connect in any logical way. It might sound like this: "I went to sit in the chair and the balloon is there because of the traffic signal." Ideas shift from one subject to another in a completely unrelated way. The thinking process is "loose" instead of being tightly ordered and logical.

In both tangentiality and loosening of associations, the disorganized thoughts come across as confused and confusing. Other problems with the ability to think clearly include poverty of content of speech and thought blocking:

- **Poverty of content of speech:** This means that what one is talking about may seem unclear, meaningless, or vague. For example, a person may have the same answer for every question asked, or have very little to say. This is similar to the negative symptom of slow or empty thinking and speech.
- **Thought blocking:** Thought blocking happens when there is an interruption in the train of thought and the person cannot put his or her thoughts into words. The thoughts are "blocked" from coming out. So, the person may be very slow to respond to questions or may not be able to respond at all. At other times, rather than actual thought blocking, the person may be too distracted to respond, such as if they are hearing voices and can't pay attention to both the voices and you at the same time.

Other forms of disorganized speech may include using words incorrectly, using new words that do not really have a recognized meaning, or using words because of what they sound like rather than because of their meanings.

Mental health professionals sometimes use the term *formal thought disorder*, or just *thought disorder*, instead of disorganization. (When those terms are used, they are usually meant to be the same as disorganization, which is a symptom of a psychotic disorder, rather than being a separate disorder themselves.) Formal thought disorder means that the difficulty is with the form of thoughts (how the person thinks) rather than with the content of thought (what the person is thinking about). That is, the form of thoughts might seem out of order, new words might be made up and used, the person's speech might be hard to follow or not make sense (like in loosening of associations), or the person might go off on tangents (as in tangentiality).

In addition to these types of disorganized thoughts and speech, individuals with psychosis may also have **disorganized behavior**. Disorganized behavior often appears as an inability to follow through with plans. It may also be seen as having a bizarre appearance, such as having shoes on the wrong feet or wearing clothes inside out. People may dress inappropriately for the weather, wearing several layers of clothing even in warm temperatures. Behavior may also become disorganized because one's thoughts are disorganized.

Impaired Insight

Unfortunately, **impaired insight** (often referred to as **unawareness of illness**) is a common experience for people with psychosis. Because their unusual experiences may be very real to them, people experiencing psychosis do not realize that the thoughts and behaviors they are having are a change from their normal self. They also may be unaware that their behavior is different from that of other people. People with impaired insight might refuse to take medicine or follow up with treatment because they simply don't see or recognize a need for it.

Impaired insight is one of the biggest challenges in psychosis, especially for family members who desperately want their loved ones to understand the illness and realize the benefits of treatment. Healthcare providers try to teach people with psychosis about their symptoms (sometimes called psychoeducation) so that their insight will improve. This helps them to engage in, or stick with, their treatment (see Chapter 9, "Follow-Up and Sticking with Treatment") and leads to better outcomes for their illness.

> Healthcare providers try to teach people with psychosis about their symptoms (sometimes called psychoeducation) so that their insight will improve. This helps them to engage in, or stick with, their treatment and leads to better outcomes for their illness.

Cognitive Dysfunction

The term **cognitive dysfunction** refers to symptoms that cause difficulties with some of the most important mental functions, like concentration, learning, memory, and planning. Although people with psychosis typically have normal or close to normal intelligence or IQ (intelligence quotient), they may have some difficulties with specific cognitive abilities, like the ability to understand, process, and recall information. Everyone has problems remembering things or paying attention from time to time. However, people with psychosis have more serious problems that are often long-lasting, especially if symptoms go untreated for a long period.

The forms of cognitive dysfunction that are part of psychosis may include difficulties with abstract thinking, poor attention and concentration, impaired information processing, poor memory, and difficulties with planning. These frequently go along with negative symptoms. Even though cognitive dysfunction often goes unnoticed, it tends to cause difficulties at school or work. Psychologists and other mental health professionals assess for cognitive dysfunction using a group of **cognitive tests**, also referred to as **neurocognitive tests** or **neuropsychological tests**. Such tests might include giving the meaning of metaphors, having to follow a series of numbers or letters on a computer screen, having to spell things backward, addition and subtraction, seeing how well things are remembered after several minutes have passed, listing as many animals as possible in a one-minute period, completing a series of mazes, and similar tests. Although some of the tests can get difficult, they are often interesting to take part in if one has motivation to do so. Some of these tests also form the basis for a treatment of cognitive dysfunction called *cognitive remediation* (see Chapter 8), where similar cognitive tests are practiced, often in a computerized format.

- **Difficulties with abstract thinking:** People with psychosis may not be able to understand complex concepts or solve problems that require them to think through several steps. In addition, they may find it difficult to understand ideas with abstract meanings, such as metaphors, proverbs, and sayings. For example, they may not understand common phrases like "don't judge a book by its cover" or "there's no use crying over spilled milk."
- **Poor attention and concentration:** People experiencing psychosis often display limitations in attention and concentration. They may have a hard time keeping their thoughts on one idea. They also may find tasks that require them to focus their attention to be very tiring. For example, they

may find it difficult to stay focused on a book or a television show for more than a few minutes.

- **Impaired information processing:** People experiencing this symptom may have difficulty sorting out information and discovering meaning in things that they observe. It may appear that things do not "sink in" the way they used to or that complex concepts seem more difficult for them to understand than before.
- **Poor memory:** People experiencing poor memory usually have trouble learning and remembering new things. Some also may have trouble remembering past events, but this is much less common.
- **Difficulties with planning:** Cognitive difficulties that occur with psychosis may make it hard to plan and follow through with plans. People may have trouble focusing on future events in a logical way. They also may not have the ability to correctly judge different plans of action. In addition, they may become uncertain and have difficulty making a decision or committing to a plan.

Hostile/Aggressive Symptoms

Most people experiencing psychosis are not dangerous or violent in any way, and the rate of violence in people experiencing psychosis is very similar to that of the population as a whole. However, some people with psychosis do show increased **hostility** or **aggression**. They may argue more than normal, destroy property, or make threats toward others. Although rare, when these behaviors do occur, they can be driven by specific delusions. For example, someone with a paranoid delusion may act out of fear, believing that they must do something for protection and safety.

Catatonic and Movement Symptoms

Catatonia is a rare syndrome that can happen together with the syndrome of psychosis. It is a severe change from normal body movements that happens without a clear reason. For example, those who have catatonia may lose the ability to move, appearing frozen, stiff, and motionless. They also may appear completely unresponsive to their environment. People with psychosis may experience less extreme movement symptoms such as moving very slowly or maintaining unnatural poses. Catatonia can be dangerous because it can keep the person from getting adequate hydration and nutrition, taking care of their hygiene, and taking medicine. In some instances, it can also cause a dangerous elevation in vital signs, such as blood pressure.

Sometimes antipsychotic medicines, especially the older "conventional" medicines, may cause movement side effects that mimic the symptoms of catatonia. But, in this case, the movement side effects (like slowness, stiffness, or tremor) are an unwanted effect of the medicines. Catatonia, on the other hand, consists of movement symptoms that are caused not by medicine but by the illness itself.

Mood Symptoms and Anxiety

Some people with a psychotic disorder may experience or express emotions less deeply, as described earlier (anhedonia, apathy, and blunted or flat affect); for others, psychosis can cause other types of changes in their mood. Some of these symptoms may be like the ones seen in other mental illnesses, such as major depression or bipolar disorder. So, it is possible that some people with psychosis may have prominent negative symptoms and a decreased expression of emotions, and others may have few or no negative symptoms but have some symptoms commonly seen in depression. Yet others may have some of the mood symptoms often seen in mania, the syndrome that occurs in bipolar disorder (see Chapter 3).

Changes in one's moods or feelings may come before psychosis, occur during a first episode of psychosis, or come after a psychotic episode. For instance, some people may experience a depressed mood, or depression. They may feel down, unhappy, or empty.

On the other hand, people with psychosis also may experience a syndrome called mania, or periods in which they feel abnormally happy, high, energetic, or excited. An exaggerated sense of self-worth, belief that one has special powers, and reckless or dangerous behaviors may also be seen in mania. Some people have a "labile affect" in which their mood quickly moves between happy and sad, such as laughing that quickly switches to crying. When someone repeatedly smiles or laughs out of context, this is called an "inappropriate affect."

It is also common for people experiencing psychosis to be anxious or nervous. One source of **anxiety** may be delusional thoughts. For example, thinking that people are following you would make anyone very anxious. Anxiety may show up in some people as being tense or jittery, worrying that something bad is going to happen, or appearing generally uneasy in most situations.

Suicidal Thoughts

People experiencing psychosis may have thoughts about dying. This may include wishing to be dead, as well as thinking about or planning to commit suicide. **Suicidal thoughts** (also called **suicidal ideation**) may be driven by several symptoms, including emotional distress due to the frightening experience of psychosis or as a direct result of hallucinations or delusions. For example, a person may hear voices instructing him or her to commit suicide (called **command hallucinations**).

In addition, people who have some level of insight into how they have changed may become hopeless and depressed. Suicidal thoughts may also happen if individuals become aware that they may not be able to achieve goals as they had planned. People with psychosis are at a much higher risk for suicide attempts and completed suicide than the population as a whole. Family and friends should, therefore, take any expression of suicidal thoughts very seriously. Ideally, specialized care for early psychosis that focuses on the individual's goals—and how to achieve them in the context of ongoing treatment and recovery—will help him or her move past suicidal thoughts.

Prodromal Symptoms

When mental health professionals speak of **prodromal symptoms**, they are talking about subtle changes in thoughts, feelings, or behaviors that happened *before* the first episode of psychosis. The prodromal period may last from a few days to a few years. Some people with psychosis may not have had any prodromal symptoms at all.

Prodromal symptoms are often similar to psychotic symptoms, just in a milder form. For example, the young person may be very suspicious but not to the extent of having paranoid delusions. A person may mistake one object for another, such as seeing spots on a wall as crawling bugs. Although this is a mistake, it is not a full hallucination because the person's mind is misinterpreting a real object. In the case of hallucinations, people are sensing or experiencing something that is not really there.

Other prodromal symptoms may be more similar to depression or anxiety than psychosis. For example, prodromal symptoms may include anxiety, declining performance in school or on the job, depressed mood, difficulty sleeping, irritability, and pulling away from significant others. Even though prodromal symptoms happened in the past, it is still important to understand them. This is because the same prodromal symptoms that happened before psychosis first began are often the same subtle symptoms that occur before another episode of psychosis. They can thus be early warning signs (as discussed in Chapter 10, "Knowing Your Early Warning Signs and Preventing a Relapse") for a worsening or return of illness (**relapse**).

> Understanding the various symptoms of psychosis, and the treatments that are most effective for them, is key to engaging in treatment and recovery. Symptoms of psychosis can be very scary for those experiencing them and for their families and friends. But help is available.

Putting It All Together

Understanding the various symptoms of psychosis, and the treatments that are most effective for them, is key to engaging in treatment and recovery. Symptoms of psychosis can be very scary for those experiencing them and for their families and friends. But help is available. People experiencing symptoms may not understand their illness or may have impaired insight. They also may despair and start to lose hope when experiencing an episode. Family and friends should take any indications of suicidal thoughts very seriously as people with psychosis are at a greater risk for attempting and completing suicide than others.

Milder symptoms experienced before the first episode of psychosis are known as prodromal symptoms. An individual's prodromal symptoms are important to remember because they usually are the same ones that occur before another episode (as such, they are early warning signs). Symptoms, whether in the past or present, are important to discuss with your mental health professional. Family members and friends are crucial sources of information for mental health professionals. In the same way, mental health professionals are very important sources of information for young people with psychosis, family members, and friends. Sharing information and making shared treatment decisions are key to successful treatment. Not only can family and friends provide information to mental health professionals about symptoms and behaviors, but they also can report how symptoms are changing over time, including when they are improving or getting worse. Mental health professionals can explain symptoms to families and report on the changes that they are seeing.

Family members and friends are crucial sources of information for mental health professionals. In the same way, mental health professionals are very important sources of information for young people with psychosis, family members, and friends. Sharing information and making shared treatment decisions are key to successful treatment.

Worksheet 2.1 can help young people with psychosis and their family members record and keep track of the symptoms that were experienced in the past or that are currently present. It is also a place to keep comments and questions that you want to discuss with your mental health professional. A printable version is available at www.oup.com/firstepisodepsychosis.

Worksheet 2.1 Symptoms Checklist	
Here is a place to identify the symptoms you have experienced. Check which symptoms have occurred and when they happened. Record any questions or comments you may have.	
Positive Symptoms	✓
Hallucinations	
Questions or Comments:	
Delusions	
Questions or Comments:	
Suspiciousness/Paranoia	
Questions or Comments:	
Ideas of Reference	
Questions or Comments:	
Bizarre Behavior	
Questions or Comments:	
Negative Symptoms	✓
Anhedonia/Loss of Interests	
Questions or Comments:	
Apathy/Not Caring as Deeply	
Questions or Comments:	

Blunted or Flat Affect	
Questions or Comments:	
Emotional Withdrawal	
Questions or Comments:	
Low Drive or Motivation	
Questions or Comments:	
Poor Grooming/Hygiene	
Questions or Comments:	
Slow or Empty Thinking and Speech	
Questions or Comments:	
Slow Movements	
Questions or Comments:	
Social Isolation	
Questions or Comments:	
Disorganization	✓
Tangentiality/Loosening of Associations	
Questions or Comments:	
Poverty of Speech Content	
Questions or Comments:	
Thought Blocking	
Questions or Comments:	
Disorganized Behavior	
Questions or Comments:	
Self-Awareness/Insight	✓
Impaired Insight	
Questions or Comments:	
Cognitive Dysfunction	✓

Difficulties with Abstract Thinking	
Questions or Comments:	
Poor Attention and Concentration	
Questions or Comments:	
Impaired Information Processing	
Questions or Comments:	
Difficulties with Memory	
Questions or Comments:	
Difficulties with Planning	
Questions or Comments:	
Aggressiveness	✓
Increased Hostility or Aggression	
Questions or Comments:	
Catatonic and Movement Symptoms	✓
Catatonia	
Questions or Comments:	
Abnormal Movements or Posturing	
Questions or Comments:	
Mood Symptoms and Suicidal Thoughts	✓
Depression	
Questions or Comments:	
Manic Symptoms	
Questions or Comments:	
Anxiety	
Questions or Comments:	
Suicidal Thoughts or Behaviors	
Questions or Comments:	

Key Chapter Points

- Like many other mental illnesses, early psychosis is a syndrome that causes many different symptoms. Different people experiencing psychosis have different types of symptoms, and a person's symptoms may change during his or her illness.
- The "positive symptoms" (called that because they are *added on* to normal experience) include hallucinations (especially hearing voices), delusions, suspiciousness/paranoia, and ideas of reference.
- The "negative symptoms" (called that because they are *taken away* from normal experience) include anhedonia; apathy; blunted affect or flat affect; emotional withdrawal; low drive, energy, or motivation; poor attention to grooming and hygiene; slow or empty thinking and speech; slow movements; and social isolation.
- Other types of symptoms include disorganized symptoms, impaired insight, cognitive dysfunction, hostile/aggressive symptoms, catatonic and movement symptoms, mood symptoms and anxiety, and even suicidal thoughts.
- Even though prodromal symptoms happened in the past, it is still important to understand them. This is because the same prodromal symptoms that happened before psychosis first began are often the same subtle symptoms that occur before another episode of psychosis. They can thus be early warning signs for a worsening or return of illness (relapse).
- Symptoms, whether in the past or present, are important to discuss with your mental health professional. Family members and friends are crucial sources of information for mental health professionals. In the same way, mental health professionals are very important sources of information for young people with psychosis, family members, and friends.

3

What Diagnoses Are Associated with Psychosis?

As described in Chapter 1 ("What Is Psychosis?"), psychosis is a syndrome. And as then detailed in Chapter 2 ("What Are the Symptoms of Psychosis?"), this syndrome can include a number of different symptoms. Different people with a first episode of psychosis have different sets of symptoms. In this chapter, we discuss the different diagnoses that may relate to psychosis. A **diagnosis** is a specific medical term given to an illness or syndrome by healthcare providers. When a psychiatrist or other mental health professional evaluates someone experiencing psychosis, he or she gathers as much information as possible. This information comes from a detailed psychiatric interview and observations, medical records, additional information from family members, a physical exam, cognitive tests, lab tests, and other types of evaluations to determine the illness underlying the episode of psychosis (see Chapter 6, "The Initial Evaluation of Psychosis").

> When a psychiatrist or other mental health professional evaluates someone experiencing psychosis, he or she gathers as much information as possible. This information comes from a detailed psychiatric interview and observations, medical records, additional information from family members, a physical exam, cognitive tests, lab tests, and other types of evaluations to determine the illness underlying the episode of psychosis.

While gathering information to evaluate a first episode of psychosis, the psychiatrist or other mental health professional often comes up with a **differential diagnosis**. This is a list of the most likely diagnoses for the syndrome, in this case psychosis. Healthcare providers generally use a differential diagnosis to list the possible illnesses underlying any health problem. For example, if you go to the doctor for a fever, the doctor may make a list of possible reasons for the fever, such as a minor cold caused by a virus, strep throat caused by bacteria, pneumonia, the flu, or other infections. To narrow down this list to the most likely diagnosis, the doctor then uses information from the history (asking questions), physical exam, and lab tests. Often healthcare providers use a **working diagnosis** (the most likely diagnosis given the available information) to guide treatment planning even if they have yet to decide on a final diagnosis

It is important for young people and families to recognize that making a specific diagnosis frequently requires long-term information that often is not fully available when a person first comes in for treatment. Being unsure about the diagnosis is one reason why a differential diagnosis and a working diagnosis are used in the short term. A working diagnosis allows the healthcare provider to begin an effective treatment plan even though a final diagnosis may not yet be clear. The symptoms of psychosis can be effectively treated without having a specific diagnosis with certainty. This chapter focuses on the three categories that are commonly part of the differential diagnosis of first-episode psychosis. Psychiatrists and other mental health professionals think through these different possible diagnoses—and conduct a thorough evaluation—before determining the one that is most likely.

> A working diagnosis allows the healthcare provider to begin an effective treatment plan even though a final diagnosis may not yet be clear. The symptoms of psychosis can be effectively treated without having a specific diagnosis with certainty.

Three Causes of Psychotic Symptoms

It is important to understand what causes the symptoms of psychosis. If the cause of the psychotic symptoms can be determined, the psychiatrist or other mental health professional can decide what treatment is best. The three main categories of causes of psychosis are (1) medical causes, (2) substances, and (3) psychiatric illnesses. We briefly describe each of these types of causes in the following pages.

Medical Causes of Psychosis

In rare instances, a physical health condition can cause psychosis. This is called a *psychotic disorder due to another medical condition*. In this diagnosis, a medical condition directly causes hallucinations or delusions. Several physical health conditions can cause psychotic symptoms. To find out if such a medical condition is causing the psychosis, the healthcare providers will do a number of things. First, they will ask questions about the young person's physical health. Then, they will do a physical exam or refer the person for one to be done. They also may do lab tests and other types of tests.

One example of a physical health problem that may cause psychosis is certain types of epilepsy, or seizure disorder. To find out if someone has a seizure disorder, the doctor will ask about certain types of symptoms and when and how they occur. Then a doctor will do a physical exam to check for signs of a neurological condition. If the doctor believes that a seizure disorder may be causing the psychosis, he or she will recommend that the young person get an electroencephalogram, or EEG. If the EEG shows a possible seizure disorder, then the doctor may conclude that this medical condition is a likely cause of the psychosis. A neurologist would then treat that condition.

Figure 3.1 lists some of the medical conditions that can sometimes cause psychosis. Some of the medical conditions that are most commonly associated with psychosis are endocrine disorders (like Addison's disease and Cushing's disease, which can affect cortisol levels in the blood), metabolic disorders (like kidney disease or liver diseases), autoimmune disorders (like lupus and the more recently recognized N-methyl-D-aspartate [NMDA] receptor autoimmune encephalitis), and temporal lobe epilepsy. Although some of the conditions listed in Figure 3.1 are more common (such as HIV/AIDS, lupus,

| Addison's disease |
| Brain infection |
| Brain tumor |
| Cushing's disease |
| Epilepsy |
| Fluid or electrolyte imbalance |
| HIV/AIDS |
| Huntington's disease |
| Hypoxia |
| Kidney diseases |
| Liver diseases |
| Multiple sclerosis |
| Neurosyphilis |
| Parathyroid diseases (hyperparathyroidism or hypoparathyroidism) |
| Parkinson's disease |
| Stroke |
| Systemic lupus erythematosus (Lupus) |
| Temporal lobe epilepsy |
| Thyroid disease (hyperthyroidism or hypothyroidism) |

Figure 3.1 Some of the Medical Conditions That Can Sometimes Cause Psychosis

and thyroid disease) than some of the others, it is very rare for them to cause psychosis. On the other hand, some are much rarer illnesses (like NMDA receptor autoimmune encephalitis), but when they do occur, they are quite likely to cause psychosis.

Although it is fairly rare for a first episode of psychosis in a young person to be caused by any of the medical conditions, it is important for doctors to rule out these medical conditions because if the psychosis is in fact due to one of these disorders, very specific medical treatments may be needed. For example, doctors use an antibiotic, such as penicillin, to treat neurosyphilis, and an anticonvulsant medicine, which prevents seizures, to treat temporal lobe epilepsy. If there is no evidence that a medical condition is causing the symptoms, then the doctor will decide whether the psychosis might be caused by substances, or if it stems from a psychiatric disorder.

Psychosis Caused by Substances

Psychosis caused by a drug or medicine is called a *substance/medication-induced psychotic disorder*. Many substances can cause psychotic symptoms. Between 7% and 25% of young people with a first episode of psychosis in different studies are reported as having substance/medication-induced psychotic disorder. To find out if a substance is causing psychosis, the healthcare provider will ask about the young person's use of certain substances and do lab tests to see if these are present in the individual's body. Figure 3.2 lists some of the addictive substances (drugs) that can sometimes cause psychosis. Other drugs, such as alcohol or addictive anxiety/sleeping pills, can cause psychosis during withdrawal from the drug.

Cocaine
Ketamine
Lysergic acid diethylamide (LSD)
Marijuana
Methamphetamine / amphetamines
Phencyclidine (PCP)
Synthetic cannabinoids

Figure 3.2 Some of the Drugs That Can Cause Psychosis

In addition to these addictive drugs, some medicines can cause psychosis. For example, medical steroids, such as prednisone (Deltasone) and dexamethasone (Decadron), may rarely cause psychosis. Methylphenidate (Ritalin), which is a treatment for attention-deficit/hyperactivity disorder usually in children and adolescents, may cause psychosis at high doses. A number of other medicines, including some of the ones used to treat HIV/AIDS, Parkinson's disease, and some other diseases, may cause psychosis in rare instances.

If a lab test (a blood test or a urine test) shows that one or more of these substances is in the young person's body, then the healthcare provider will recommend that he or she stop using these substances. If a medicine appears to be causing the psychosis, the psychiatrist or other mental health professional will work with the young person's medical doctor to change the medicine. It may take several days for the substance or medicine to wash out of the person's body. If the substance is causing the psychosis, the psychotic symptoms will usually go away when it is gone from the body. If the substance is not causing the psychosis, the psychotic symptoms will continue even when the substance is gone. When neither a medical condition nor substance use appears to be causing the psychotic symptoms, the psychiatrist or other mental health professional may decide that the young person's symptoms are most likely psychiatric in origin.

It can sometimes be very challenging to determine whether the psychosis is drug induced or caused by a psychiatric disorder. Some substances, such as marijuana, may be partly responsible for the onset of psychosis even though the symptoms do not go away when the substance is no longer present (see Chapter 4, "What Causes Primary Psychotic Disorders Like Schizophrenia?"). Thus, it is often unclear whether substance use is a trigger for a primary psychotic disorder such as schizophrenia (see next section) or whether the illness is a substance/medication-induced psychotic disorder. Nonetheless, it is possible to start effective treatment for psychosis without making a specific diagnosis with certainty. The diagnosis usually becomes clearer as some time passes.

Psychiatric Causes of Psychosis

When neither a medical condition nor substance use appears to be causing the psychotic symptoms, the psychiatrist or other mental health professional may decide that the young person's symptoms are most likely psychiatric in origin. This means that the symptoms are coming from a brain disturbance and are usually best understood by, and treated by, psychiatrists and other mental health professionals. At this time, there are no lab tests or other medical tests that can prove a psychiatric disorder. So, unlike detecting a medical condition through a medical test or finding a substance in one's body through a urine or blood test, the evaluation of psychiatric disorders depends heavily on a detailed interview and observations. That is, the mental health professional talks to the young person about recent symptoms and gathers information from his or her family about changes in feelings, thoughts, and behaviors. Several types of psychiatric illnesses can lead to the syndrome of psychosis, so the mental health professional will develop a differential diagnosis, or the most likely diagnoses for the psychosis (see Table 3.1). He or she may need to decide on a working diagnosis before a final diagnosis becomes clear.

Mental health professionals use two sources for classifying psychiatric disorders. One is the ***Diagnostic and Statistical Manual of Mental Disorders* (DSM)**, which is currently in its fifth edition. The other is the **International Classification of Diseases (ICD)**, which is currently in its 10th edition. Both the DSM and the ICD provide specific definitions of psychiatric disorders. This allows all healthcare providers to consistently use the same diagnostic terminology when referring to a specific syndrome. As a result, DSM and ICD provide consistent definitions for psychiatric illnesses around the world. So, for example, the definition for schizophrenia is the same in North America,

Table 3.1 Diagnoses Associated with Psychosis

Psychotic Disorder Due to Another Medical Condition	(see Figure 3.1)
Substance/Medication-Induced Psychotic Disorder	(see Figure 3.2)
Primary Psychotic Disorders	Brief psychotic disorder Schizophreniform disorder Schizophrenia Schizoaffective disorder Delusional disorder Other specified schizophrenia spectrum and other psychotic disorder Unspecified schizophrenia spectrum and other psychotic disorder
Other Disorders that May Cause Psychosis or Psychotic-Like Symptoms	Postpartum psychosis Major depression Bipolar disorder Schizotypal personality disorder (or Schizotypal disorder) Delirium Dementia

Europe, and Australia. This is especially important because the exact causes of most psychiatric illnesses are still unclear. So, rather than defining a mental illness by the exact cause, mental health professionals use symptoms to classify the illness. Next, we describe a number of psychiatric disorders, based on definitions found in the DSM-5.

Primary Psychotic Disorders

One group of psychiatric disorders that causes psychosis are the **primary psychotic disorders**. They are called this because they primarily cause psychosis, rather than depression, anxiety, or another type of syndrome. The most common of these is schizophrenia, followed by other disorders closely related to schizophrenia. The seven primary psychotic disorders are (1) brief psychotic disorder, (2) schizophreniform disorder, (3) schizophrenia, (4) schizoaffective disorder, (5) delusional disorder, (6) other specified schizophrenia spectrum and other psychotic disorder, and (7) unspecified schizophrenia spectrum and other psychotic disorder.

Brief Psychotic Disorder

People diagnosed with brief psychotic disorder have one or more positive symptoms (hallucinations or delusions) or disorganized speech or behavior, but these symptoms last only up to one month. Functioning then returns to normal and symptoms go away. Brief psychotic disorder may sometimes happen after a very stressful event, such as the exposure to a serious natural disaster or being in war or combat. This disorder is uncommon, but when it does happen, it is most likely to happen when a person is between the ages of 20 and 40 years. While someone with a brief psychotic disorder has similar symptoms to schizophrenia, the symptoms clear up rapidly and do not return. It is a single psychotic episode that does not recur. If psychosis does return, then the diagnosis will most likely be changed to one of those described later in this section.

Schizophreniform Disorder

People diagnosed with schizophreniform disorder have a combination of psychotic symptoms that last at least one month, and up to six months. The combination of symptoms includes two or more of the following: delusions, hallucinations, disorganized speech, disorganized or catatonic behavior, and negative symptoms (see Chapter 2). Schizophreniform disorder is a psychotic episode that lasts longer than brief psychotic disorder, but does not last long enough to receive a diagnosis of schizophrenia. If the symptoms last for longer than six months, then the diagnosis is changed from schizophreniform disorder to schizophrenia or one of the other primary psychotic disorders. In this way, individuals ultimately diagnosed with schizophrenia may have received the diagnosis of schizophreniform disorder during the first six months of the illness.

Schizophrenia

People with schizophrenia have a combination of psychotic symptoms. Specifically, schizophrenia is defined by the presence of two or more of the following: delusions, hallucinations, disorganized speech, disorganized or catatonic behavior, and negative symptoms, and the illness lasts for longer than six months. So, schizophrenia is very similar to schizophreniform disorder except that in schizophrenia, symptoms last longer. In fact, schizophrenia usually lasts for a very long time and may even be lifelong. People with schizophrenia often need some form of treatment long term. When a person with schizophrenia continues with his or her treatment (see Chapter 9, "Follow-up and Sticking with Treatment"), the symptoms often do not get worse and may get much better. In fact, the positive symptoms often respond quite well to treatment. Many people who continue treatment are able to have good lives with steady jobs and happy relationships, which is the goal of the **recovery model** (see Chapter 12, "Embracing Recovery"). The recovery model of mental health treatment aims to empower the individual to achieve his or her own goals for recovery by actively participating in treatment decisions.

People all over the world have schizophrenia. About 1 in every 100 persons develops schizophrenia during their lifetime. In other words, over the course of one's lifetime, the risk of having schizophrenia is about 1%. Schizophrenia affects men and women approximately equally, though it may be slightly more common in men. The symptoms of schizophrenia usually first become apparent in men between the ages of about 20 and 30, and in women between the ages of about 24 and 34. However, people who are younger or older also may develop the illness. In fact, "childhood-onset schizophrenia" has been defined by some as the development of the illness before age 12, and "late-onset schizophrenia" is considered to be the development of the illness after age 40.

At first, family and friends may think that someone developing psychotic symptoms is "going through a phase." They may not notice the earliest symptoms. But after a while, the symptoms become more obvious. For example, the person may have unusual beliefs, no longer be interested in work or school, have outbursts of anger, stop bathing regularly, or talk to himself or herself due to hearing voices.

Schizoaffective Disorder

People with schizoaffective disorder have a combination of psychotic symptoms and serious mood symptoms. The mood symptoms may be like the symptoms seen in clinical depression, also called major depression, or they may be like the symptoms seen in mania, or bipolar disorder. So, there are two types of schizoaffective disorder:

- In **schizoaffective disorder—depressive type**, the person has the symptoms of schizophrenia described earlier, but also at times has symptoms of **depression**. These may include feeling sad or depressed, not being as interested in fun or pleasurable things, a decreased or increased appetite, weight loss or weight gain, having difficulty sleeping or sleeping too much, feeling agitated, feeling slow, fatigue, loss of energy, feeling worthless, feeling guilty for no apparent reason, having difficulty concentrating or making decisions, or having thoughts of death or thoughts of committing suicide.
- In **schizoaffective disorder—bipolar type**, the person has the symptoms of schizophrenia, but also at times has symptoms of **mania**. These may include thinking too highly of oneself (an inflated self-esteem, also called grandiosity), not needing to sleep due to having enough energy without sleep, being more talkative than usual, talking very rapidly, having racing thoughts, having poor attention, being agitated, engaging in many different activities, or going on spending sprees.

Schizoaffective disorder is less common than schizophrenia. It can start at any age, but most often starts in a person's 20s or 30s, like schizophrenia. Like in schizophrenia, many people with schizoaffective disorder who continue treatment are able to have good lives, jobs, and relationships, which are the goals of treatment that follows the recovery model.

Delusional Disorder

Delusional disorder is similar to schizophrenia, except the main symptom is a single delusion. For example, the person may be convinced that a famous person is in love with them, that someone is following or out to get them, or that a medical condition is present when in fact it is not. Delusional disorder is quite rare, but when it does happen, it tends to be somewhat less severe than schizophrenia or schizoaffective disorder because many of the other types of symptoms that may occur with schizophrenia or schizoaffective disorder (like hallucinations, disorganized thinking, negative symptoms, and cognitive dysfunction) are not present.

Other Specified Schizophrenia Spectrum and Other Psychotic Disorder

Although the name of this diagnosis is confusing, it means that the symptoms of a primary psychotic disorder (like schizophrenia) are present, but the "full criteria" for any of the preceding five psychotic disorders are not met. Mental health professionals making this diagnosis can then "specify" further what is meant. For example, the person might have ongoing, serious auditory hallucinations, but does not have the other symptoms required for a diagnosis of schizophrenia. Another example is when a close relative of someone with delusional disorder might also have some of the same delusional thoughts, but does not meet full criteria for delusional disorder themselves.

Unspecified Schizophrenia Spectrum and Other Psychotic Disorder

People given this diagnosis also have symptoms of a primary psychotic disorder (like schizophrenia), but again do not meet the full criteria for any of the five primary psychotic disorders. Mental health professionals using this diagnosis do not specify further details. This diagnosis is most often used when there is not yet enough information to make one of the five specific diagnoses described earlier. That is, mental health professionals often use this as a preliminary diagnosis before deciding on a more conclusive diagnosis once more information is obtained. Sometimes a person may receive a new, updated diagnosis when more is learned about their symptoms and a more detailed evaluation can be conducted.

Other Psychiatric Disorders That Can Cause Psychosis

Several other disorders can bring about psychotic symptoms (or symptoms that are very similar to psychotic symptoms). These disorders include post-partum psychosis, major depressive disorder, bipolar disorder, schizotypal personality disorder (or schizotypal disorder), delirium, and dementia.

Psychiatrists and other mental health professionals give a diagnosis of **post-partum psychosis** when a woman has psychotic symptoms anytime within the first three months after giving birth. The symptoms usually begin within the first month after the child's birth and usually come on fairly suddenly. Unlike postpartum depression, which involves depressive symptoms, post-partum psychosis involves having psychotic symptoms, like hallucinations or delusions. Postpartum psychosis usually gets better with treatment.

Major depression, also called major depressive disorder or clinical depres-sion, is when one has been experiencing multiple symptoms of depression for at least two weeks. A depressive episode may last weeks, months, or even years. Symptoms may include those listed earlier related to schizoaffective disorder—depressive type. These symptoms of depression are feeling sad or depressed, not being as interested in fun or pleasurable things, a decreased or increased appetite, weight loss or weight gain, having difficulty sleeping, sleeping too much, feeling agitated, feeling slow, fatigue, loss of energy, feeling worthless, feeling guilty for no apparent reason, having difficulty con-centrating or making decisions, or having thoughts of death or thoughts of committing suicide.

Major depression is a common psychiatric disorder—much more common than schizophrenia and other primary psychotic disorders. Whereas schizo-phrenia affects about 1% of people over the course of their lifetime, an episode of major depression may occur in as many as one in four (25% or one-fourth) of all people during their lifetime. In most cases, major depression does not cause psychosis. However, in some instances, when the depression becomes severe, psychotic symptoms may develop. This is called *psychotic depres-sion*. The psychosis usually clears up and goes away altogether when the in-dividual receives adequate treatment for depression. Such treatments usually include medicines called **antidepressants**, as well as one of several types of psychotherapy.

A mental health professional gives a diagnosis of **bipolar disorder** when someone has had one or more episodes of mania. Episodes of major depres-sion may happen in between the episodes of mania. As listed earlier in the description of schizoaffective disorder—bipolar type, symptoms of mania may include thinking too highly of oneself (an inflated self-esteem, also called grandiosity), not needing to sleep due to having enough energy without sleep, being more talkative than usual, talking very rapidly, having racing thoughts, having poor attention, being agitated, engaging in many different activities, or going on spending sprees. Like major depression, many cases of mania do not cause psychotic symptoms. However, when the manic episode is severe, psychotic symptoms like hallucinations or delusions may develop. Also, like psychotic depression, once the mania is adequately treated, the psychosis usually clears up and goes away. Treatments for bipolar disorder include medicines, some of which are **mood stabilizers**, as well as certain types of psychotherapy. Distinguishing between bipolar disorder with psychosis and schizoaffective disorder—bipolar type is sometimes difficult. Often, a working diagnosis is made, and then once more long-term observation and monitoring is available, it becomes clearer whether the young person's symptoms are more consistent with bipolar disorder or schizoaffective disorder.

Mental health professionals think of **schizotypal personality disorder** (also called schizotypal disorder) as a mild form of schizophrenia that never leads to the full syndrome of psychosis. A person with this diagnosis may have strange beliefs or odd behaviors, or be socially withdrawn or uncomfortable with close relationships. The person has had such symptoms or behaviors since he or she was young, and they seem to just be part of their personality. The person may seem odd and eccentric, but the symptoms are not true psychosis.

Both **delirium** and **dementia** are disorders that cause confusion and **disorientation**. That is, people with either of these conditions may not know the date, where they are, or even their name. People with primary psychotic disorders like schizophrenia, or any of the other disorders described earlier, usually do not have this form of confusion or disorientation; they know who they are, where they are, and what the date is.

Delirium is a state of confusion that develops rapidly, over the course of hours or days. It is usually due to a medical condition, like having had a seizure, having a high fever, or having an infection somewhere in the body. Delirium may also be caused by drug use or withdrawing from some drugs, like alcohol. Delirium is a medical emergency requiring immediate medical attention to treat the underlying cause of the delirium. Delirium can happen in people of any age but is more common among older people. In addition to causing confusion, delirium can sometimes cause psychotic symptoms, like hallucinations.

Dementia also causes confusion and disorientation, but dementia usually develops slowly, over the course of months or years. Dementia usually occurs in older people, usually after the age of 65, and often after the age of

80. The most common cause of dementia is Alzheimer's disease, though other diseases, such as repeated strokes, Parkinson's disease, or Huntington's disease, may cause dementia as well. In addition to causing confusion, dementia can sometimes cause psychotic symptoms, like hallucinations or delusions.

Putting It All Together

There are several different diagnoses associated with psychosis. The three major categories of illnesses that can bring about psychosis are those related to medical illnesses, substance use, and psychiatric illnesses. Chapter 4 discusses in detail what research has uncovered about the likely causes of primary psychotic disorders like schizophrenia.

Schizophrenia is one of several primary psychotic disorders, a group of psychiatric disorders that primarily cause psychosis. Other disorders can cause psychotic symptoms or similar symptoms, but are not considered psychotic disorders. A few examples of such disorders include major depressive disorder, bipolar disorder, and dementia. It is often difficult to make a specific diagnosis when long-term information is not available at first. In instances in which a definitive diagnosis is uncertain, a working diagnosis allows the healthcare provider to begin effective treatments for the psychosis even before a final diagnosis is made.

Key Chapter Points

- A diagnosis is a specific medical term given to an illness or syndrome by health-care providers.
- The three main categories of causes of psychosis are (1) medical causes, (2) substance use, and (3) psychiatric illnesses.
- Sometimes a specific diagnosis is difficult to make initially, so mental health professionals often use a working diagnosis in order to start a treatment plan. It is possible to start effective treatment for psychosis without having a specific diagnosis with certainty. In these cases, the diagnosis usually becomes clearer as some time passes.
- To make a diagnosis, psychiatrists and other mental health professionals use information from a detailed psychiatric interview and observations, other records and collateral information, a physical exam, cognitive tests, lab tests, and other types of evaluations.
- When deciding on the final diagnosis, mental health professionals use either of two classifications, the DSM or ICD, which give detailed, standard definitions for each psychiatric disorder.
- The five main primary psychotic disorders are brief psychotic disorder, schizophreniform disorder, schizophrenia, schizoaffective disorder, and delusional disorder.
- Other psychiatric disorders that can bring about psychotic symptoms (or symptoms that are very similar to psychotic symptoms) include postpartum psychosis, major depressive disorder, bipolar disorder, schizotypal personality disorder (or schizotypal disorder), delirium, and dementia.

4

What Causes Primary Psychotic Disorders Like Schizophrenia?

Doctors and researchers have been able to identify the causes of a variety of medical conditions, such as the common cold, a heart attack, and gout, to name a few. For example, there are different types of viruses that cause the symptoms of a common cold. By knowing what causes a medical problem, doctors are able to treat the condition in the most focused way possible. In the previous chapter, three general categories of causes of psychosis were presented: (1) medical causes, (2) substances, including certain drugs of abuse and several medicines, and (3) a number of psychiatric illnesses. This chapter describes what is currently known about the causes of the third of these, psychiatric illnesses, especially primary psychotic disorders like schizophrenia.

Some health conditions have a single, straightforward cause. For example, the common cold is caused by a virus. However, many illnesses do not have a single identifiable cause. Rather, they are caused by a combination of **risk factors**. A risk factor is any event or exposure that occurs before the illness and that research has shown plays a role in causing the illness. For example, cigarette smoking is a well-known risk factor for lung cancer. Smoking occurs before the lung cancer develops, and researchers have proven that smoking cigarettes plays a part in causing many cases of lung cancer. Because schizophrenia and related psychotic disorders are such complex illnesses, it is sometimes unclear if some of the risk factors truly occur before the illness. Some risk factors may make some people more prone to psychosis (see Chapter 1, "What Is Psychosis?"). In other words, some risk factors are best thought of as increasing one's tendency toward psychosis rather than actually causing psychosis.

Over the past several decades, researchers have identified some of the likely causes of complex medical conditions like diabetes, high blood pressure, and psychosis. For each of these, as is true of most medical conditions, there is no single cause. Rather, a number of risk factors, both internal (like certain genes) and external (like exposures that stress the body, such as stressful life events or drug use) combine in complex ways to bring about the illness. Research is showing that some genes may increase one's risk for schizophrenia only when certain external exposures are also present. For example, some research studies suggest that one particular gene that may increase risk for schizophrenia only seems to do so in people who smoked marijuana during adolescence.

Psychotic disorders are not the result of a single cause like the virus that causes the symptoms of the common cold. Instead, a combination of risk factors causes psychosis. This chapter first briefly describes the important role of genes as a cause of primary psychotic disorders like schizophrenia, and then a number of risk factors occurring early in life (during pregnancy/delivery and in infancy). The combination of certain genes and a number of these early life risk factors probably leads to subtle, even undetectable, abnormal early brain development, which sets the stage for the later development of psychosis. We then describe other risk factors that may occur during childhood and adolescence and that bring about further subtle abnormal brain development during adolescence. This combination of genes, early life risk factors, later risk factors, and subtle abnormal brain development ultimately may lead to the onset of psychosis. As explained at the end of this chapter, this way of viewing the cause of schizophrenia and related disorders is consistent with the two models discussed in Chapter 1, the neurodevelopmental model and the diathesis–stress model.

Genes

Most people with a primary psychotic disorder like schizophrenia do not have any relatives with the illness. However, research has shown that the more closely related someone is to a person with a psychotic disorder, the more likely they are to develop a similar illness. First-degree relatives of someone with psychosis (parents, siblings, and children) are more likely to also have psychosis than people who are not relatives of someone with psychosis. As mentioned in the previous chapter, the lifetime risk of developing schizophrenia is about 1%. That is, 1 in 100 people will develop schizophrenia over the course of a lifetime. For people with a first-degree relative with schizophrenia, like a mother, father, sister, or brother, this risk goes up to approximately 15%. Research also has shown that among twins, if one twin has schizophrenia, an identical twin is much more likely to also develop schizophrenia (about 50% or one-half chance) compared to a fraternal or non-identical twin (about 15% chance). This information indicates that psychosis is **heritable**, which means that it is partly caused by genes. **Genes** are segments of DNA that pass along the "blueprints" of how the body's cells make proteins. Proteins, in turn, form the building blocks for all parts of the body, including the brain.

Researchers now know that a large portion of the cause of schizophrenia, approximately 80% to 85%, comes from genes (Figure 4.1). It is unlikely that only one gene can cause psychosis. Rather, a number of genes probably each play a small role in a person's likelihood of developing psychosis. It may be the combination of a number of these **risk genes** that accounts for the genetic portion of the cause of schizophrenia. Researchers are working to determine the exact genes that increase risk for schizophrenia. To date, they have found a number of candidate genes (genes that have a strong possibility of being risk genes). For example, some of these candidate genes are genes that affect the dopamine and glutamate systems in the brain. However, more research is needed to prove which genes play a role in causing schizophrenia and which do not. Also, because genes serve as the "blueprints" for cells to make specific proteins, more research is needed to better understand the role of specific proteins in the development of the disorder.

> Researchers now know that a large portion of the cause of schizophrenia, approximately 80% to 85%, comes from genes. It is unlikely that only one gene can cause psychosis. Rather, a number of genes probably each play a small role in a person's likelihood of developing psychosis.

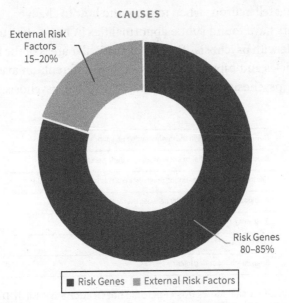

Figure 4.1 The Causes of Primary Psychotic Disorders Such as Schizophrenia

Risk Factors That Occur Before Birth, During Delivery, and in Infancy

As mentioned earlier, a number of risk factors may combine to bring about psychosis. Many of these risk factors are the risk genes that make up a large portion of the cause of psychosis. However, some risk factors are non-genetic, meaning that they are not due to one's genes. It is estimated that 15% to 20% (or about one-fifth) of the cause of schizophrenia is driven by these external risk factors. Some of these risk factors occur very early in life, before birth, during delivery, or in infancy. A few of these are shown in Figure 4.2.

Subtle Abnormalities in Early Brain Development

Researchers believe that the combination of risk genes and external risk factors that may occur early in life leads to subtle abnormalities in early brain development. These abnormalities in brain development may even occur before birth, during fetal brain development.

Genes are important in the development of the brain. They control the growth and development of cells in the brain, called **neurons**. Genes provide neurons with a "blueprint" of how to make proteins that support the structure and function of the brain. Certain genes make **neurotransmitters,** or the substances needed for communication between neurons. There are also specific genes that tell neurons when to grow and how to change.

Researchers have found subtle abnormalities in brain structure and function in people with psychosis. The size of particular areas of the brain, like the lateral ventricles and hippocampus, is slightly different, on average, in individuals with psychosis compared to those without psychosis. Studies have

| Nutritional deficiency in the mother during pregnancy |
| Exposure of the mother to a severe stressor during pregnancy |
| Infections in the mother during pregnancy (such as influenza, or the flu) |
| Rh blood-type incompatibility between the mother and fetus |
| Pregnancy and delivery complications |
| Low birth weight |
| Brain infections during infancy |

Figure 4.2 Early Life Risk Factors (Risk Factors That Occur Before Birth, During Delivery, and in Infancy)

shown that people with psychosis have abnormal patterns of activity in particular brain regions, including the frontal cortex. There also appear to be abnormalities in the neurotransmitters that allow neurons to communicate. This leads to altered communication among cells in the brain. For example, individuals with psychosis seem to have higher levels of the neurotransmitter **dopamine** in some parts of the brain and lower levels in other parts. Individuals with psychosis also have altered brain levels of other neurotransmitters, such as **glutamate**.

The abnormalities in brain development that occur early in life among people who later develop psychosis are very subtle and usually remain undetected. Ongoing research aims to be able to detect these subtle abnormalities earlier, so that someday psychosis might be preventable.

> The subtle abnormalities in early brain development early in life usually do not lead to psychosis during childhood or early adolescence. Rather, psychosis usually first begins in late adolescence or young adulthood, most often in the age range of 16 to 30 years.

Risk Factors Occurring During Childhood and Adolescence

The subtle abnormalities in early brain development early in life usually do not lead to psychosis during childhood or early adolescence. Rather, psychosis usually first begins in late adolescence or young adulthood, most often in the age range of 16 to 30 years. However, research has shown that most children who later develop schizophrenia do have some difficulties early in life. For example, they may have poor motor coordination, minor decreases in intelligence or IQ (intelligence quotient) compared to what would be expected, and subtle difficulties in social adjustment. These difficulties may lead to declining grades during middle school or high school. Children who later develop schizophrenia are also more likely to have social anxiety and other subtle psychological and social difficulties than children who do not develop schizophrenia. People who later develop psychosis also may have experienced minor psychotic-like experiences during childhood and adolescence. These are like the schizotypal or psychotic-like symptoms described in the continuum of psychosis presented in Chapter 1.

Some additional risk factors for psychosis may occur during childhood and adolescence. These risk factors may not lead to any problems in most people.

However, for those who already have early brain abnormalities because of a combination of risk genes and early life risk factors, these additional risk factors during childhood and adolescence may ultimately bring about schizophrenia. Some of these risk factors are shown in Figure 4.3. For example, various **stressful life events** may be a risk factor for schizophrenia. Such difficulties may include child abuse, discrimination, poverty, and the sense of "social defeat" that these problems may lead to.

Another external factor that may be a risk factor for schizophrenia and other primary psychotic disorders is substance use during adolescence. Research suggests that adolescent drug use, especially marijuana use, increases one's risk of developing psychosis. The main active ingredients in marijuana may affect the brain systems (for example, the dopamine neurotransmitter system) that are affected in schizophrenia. Most adolescents who use marijuana do not develop schizophrenia. However, for those with a combination of risk genes and early life risk factors, using marijuana may be a dangerous "second hit" to an already at-risk brain.

Subtle Abnormalities in Brain Development During Adolescence

Individuals who develop a psychotic disorder usually experience their first episode of psychosis between the ages of 16 and 30 years. However, some may show signs as early as middle school, while other people will not display psychotic symptoms until their 30s (and in some cases, even later).

Adolescence is an important period in the development of the brain. As the adolescent brain develops, young people experience development in social, psychological, and educational areas. Coping skills mature during this time. Many adolescents describe this period as being particularly stressful because of all the changes that come along with the move toward independence and

Child abuse

Ethnic or racial discrimination

Social adversity (such as poverty)

Marijuana use during adolescence

Figure 4.3 Risk Factors Happening During Childhood and Adolescence

adulthood. Adolescents also experience many social pressures, such as doing well in school and making friends. For someone whose genes and early life risk factors put them at risk for psychosis, these pressures may interact with normal hormonal changes of adolescence to bring about subtle brain abnormalities and problems in the dopamine system.

> Individuals who develop psychosis often display slight signs during adolescence. These signs may include mood changes, anxiety, irritability, mild positive symptoms (such as suspiciousness or odd beliefs), social withdrawal, and cognitive dysfunction. These slight signs, which make up the prodromal phase, often last several months to several years before the onset of psychosis.

Individuals who develop psychosis often display slight signs during adolescence. These signs may include mood changes, anxiety, irritability, mild positive symptoms (such as suspiciousness or odd beliefs), social withdrawal, and cognitive dysfunction. These slight signs, which make up the prodromal phase, often last a few days to a few years before the onset of psychosis (see Chapter 10, "Knowing Your Early Warning Signs and Preventing a Relapse"). People who later develop psychosis also often experience mild learning problems or school difficulties in childhood and adolescence. These are mild forms of the cognitive dysfunction (such as problems with attention, learning, memory, and planning) that are described in Chapter 2 ("What Are the Symptoms of Psychosis?").

Research suggests that in addition to the subtle abnormalities that occur in early brain development (for example, during fetal growth and infancy), additional subtle abnormalities may also occur during the important period of adolescent brain maturation. In addition to the abnormalities in neurons and neurotransmitters described earlier, other abnormalities may occur that relate to the connections between neurons. That is, a normal process of "pruning" occurs in childhood and adolescence to optimize these connections. Synaptic pruning produces more efficient connections in the brain by reducing the number of "weak" connections between neurons. Abnormalities of the pruning process during adolescent development may be under genetic control, but risk factors that happen during adolescence may also affect it.

Putting It All Together

We have described a series of events that usually occurs quietly without recognition or any idea that a primary psychotic disorder may be developing. School difficulties and social problems may develop during childhood and adolescence, so the developing illness is often not completely silent during this early stage. But these common problems would not usually prompt parents to seek psychiatric evaluation until more obvious symptoms have appeared.

This series of events includes a combination of risk genes, early life risk factors, subtle abnormalities in early brain development, risk factors during childhood and adolescence, and subtle abnormalities in brain development during adolescence. Researchers currently believe that this is the likely path toward the brain dysfunction that leads to the symptoms of psychosis.

This series of events is consistent with two models that were mentioned in Chapter 1, the neurodevelopmental model and the diathesis–stress model. That is, as shown in Figure 4.4, psychosis comes about due to a cascade of events occurring during neurodevelopment, or brain development. Also as shown in Figure 4.4, the cause of psychosis is related to both genetic risk ("diathesis") and external risk factors during childhood and adolescence ("stress").

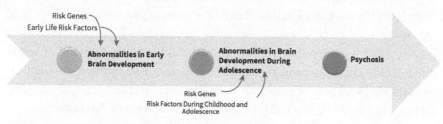

Figure 4.4 The Likely Path Toward Developing Psychosis

Key Chapter Points

- The combination of certain genes and a number of early life risk factors probably leads to subtle abnormalities in brain development, which set the stage for the later development of psychosis.
- It is unlikely that only one gene can cause psychosis. Instead, a number of genes each play a small role in a person's risk for developing psychosis.
- The abnormal brain development that happens early in life among people who later develop psychosis is very subtle and usually remains undetected and quiet.
- In addition to the subtle abnormalities in early brain development, additional subtle abnormalities may also happen during the important period of adolescent brain maturation.
- Research suggests that adolescent drug use, especially marijuana use, increases one's risk of developing psychosis.

PART II

CLARIFYING THE INITIAL EVALUATION AND TREATMENT OF PSYCHOSIS

5

Finding the Best Care

Specialty Programs for Early Psychosis

People of all ages and with different types of mental illnesses go to see a psychiatrist, take medicine, and participate in counseling with mental health professionals. They receive these services in a mental health clinic or the office of a mental health professional. Most young people with a first episode of psychosis also receive ongoing treatment in an outpatient setting like this. In some cases, this outpatient care might begin after a short stay in the hospital for the purposes of an in-depth evaluation and stabilization.

In treating a first episode of psychosis, many psychiatrists and other mental health professionals have received additional training, but this particular mental illness might not be their only focus; that is, they might see people with other mental illnesses too. However, in some places around the world, there are specialty clinics that are specifically devoted to people in the early stages of psychosis. These are sometimes called **early intervention services**. In the United States, they are sometimes called **coordinated specialty care** programs.

These specialty programs have a number of different types of mental health professionals, including psychiatrists, psychologists, nurses, social workers, counselors, employment specialists, peer specialists, and others. **Peer specialists** are individuals who themselves have gone through evaluation and treatment for a mental illness like a psychotic disorder, and who now have a job as part of the mental health team. They have a special role in assisting young people with psychosis and their family members because they have the "lived experience" of what it's like to be in treatment and to be engaged in recovery.

> Peer specialists are individuals who themselves have gone through evaluation and treatment for a mental illness like a psychotic disorder, and who now have a job as part of the mental health team. They have a special role in assisting young people with psychosis and their family members because they have the "lived experience" of what it's like to be in treatment and to be engaged in recovery.

The members of the mental health team in specialty programs for early psychosis focus on the specific needs of young people, usually between the ages of 16 and 30, who have only recently been diagnosed with a psychotic disorder. Some programs, like the Early Psychosis Prevention and Intervention Centre (EPPIC) in Melbourne, Victoria, Australia, operate within the framework of a larger youth health service. Such youth services treat many different types of mental health issues in young people. Other programs are located primarily in adult mental health services. Typically, these specialty programs provide someone with two to three years of ongoing treatment. At that point, the person is often transitioned to other outpatient care in a more general clinic setting.

Specialty programs usually do a full evaluation (see Chapter 6, "The Initial Evaluation of Psychosis") of the young person; this evaluation may have begun during a short hospital stay in some cases. The specialty programs also provide ongoing medication management as well as a number of psychosocial treatments. In addition to individual-level care, such programs may offer classes or group meetings just for young people who have recently been diagnosed with a psychotic disorder, and other group meetings for the families of these young people.

The Growth of Specialty Programs for Early Psychosis

During the past couple of decades, a number of countries—including Australia, Canada, the United Kingdom, and several countries of Western Europe, to name a few—have been providing multicomponent specialty care for early psychosis. During that time, in the United States, such services largely existed only in research centers, and were not widely available. But coordinated specialty care in the United States started becoming much more available after a large-scale study called Recovery After an Initial Schizophrenia Episode (RAISE), which was carried out from 2010 to 2014. This project was funded by the National Institute of Mental Health (NIMH) and took place in 34 clinics within 21 states. It showed effectiveness of the coordinated specialty care model compared to more traditional outpatient mental health care. That is, it was more effective in terms of better engagement of the client to the program, improved quality of life, and reduced symptoms. These programs also help young people get back into school or into a job if either of those are among the client's goals. Another RAISE project looked into best ways to establish these specialized services in outpatient clinics.

Based in part on the results of the RAISE projects, in 2014, the U.S. federal government provided an increase of 5% to the block grants that states get for mental health services. It required states to set aside 5% of their funds for evidence-based programs that address the needs of individuals with early mental illnesses, such as the first episode of psychosis. This was increased to 10% in 2016 and later. Because of these federal initiatives, coordinated specialty care programs now exist in nearly every state. Some states have several such programs in different regions of the state.

What Do Specialty Programs for Early Psychosis Provide?

Despite some differences, most specialty programs for early psychosis have a number of things in common. As mentioned earlier, many of these programs provide treatment to young people for about two to three years after they are diagnosed with a psychotic disorder. Most specialty programs for first-episode psychosis provide a combination of services, including medicines, therapy, classes, groups, case management, assistance with goals for work and school, and community outreach. The idea behind this approach is that the different pieces work best if provided together in a coordinated way tailored for the individual. The treatment plan for each individual is tailored to his or her own needs, depending on the types of symptoms present, how serious the symptoms are, and the types of other challenges going on in the young person's life.

> Most specialty programs for first-episode psychosis provide a combination of services, including medicines, therapy, classes, groups, case management, assistance with goals for work and school, and community outreach. The idea behind this approach is that the different pieces work best if provided together in a coordinated way tailored for the individual.

Coordinated Specialty Care

Specialty programs for early psychosis are sometimes called *coordinated specialty care programs*. They are recovery-oriented (see Chapter 12, "Embracing Recovery") and provide treatments proven to be effective for early psychosis. Figure 5.1 summarizes the typical parts of coordinated specialty care. The

Recovery-oriented principles of care
Helping young people with early psychosis achieve their goals for school, work, and relationships
Shared decision-making
Medication management using the lowest possible effective dosages
Individual counseling or psychotherapy
Family psychoeducation and support
Case management
Supported employment and supported education
Skills training
Screening, assessment, and treatment for substance use disorders
Screening, assessment, and treatment for suicidal thoughts or behaviors

Figure 5.1 Common Components of Early Intervention Services or Coordinated Specialty Care Programs

specialists on the team work with the client to create a personalized treatment plan using **shared decision-making**. The team offers medication management geared toward individuals with a first episode of psychosis, using the lowest dose possible, as described in Chapter 7, "Medicines Used to Treat Psychosis." The team also provides psychosocial treatments as described in Chapter 8 ("Psychosocial Treatments for Early Psychosis"), including individual psychotherapy, family psychoeducation and support, case management, help with work or school in the form of supported employment and supported education, and other treatments. Following the principles of shared decision-making, both the young person and their family have a voice in treatment decisions based on all available options.

As noted earlier, there are now many different programs that are considered coordinated specialty care in the United States, focusing on recovery, shared decision-making, and individuals' life goals. These programs also provide outreach to the community to aid in earlier detection that will hopefully reduce delays to getting into care. Just a few examples of coordinated specialty care programs include the Specialized Treatment Early in Psychosis (STEP) program at the Connecticut Mental Health Center; the Early Diagnosis and Preventive Treatment (EDAPT) program at the University of California, Davis Medical Center; the Early Assessment and Support Alliance (EASA) in Oregon; and FIRST Coordinated Specialty Care at the Department of Psychiatry at Northeast Ohio Medical University and related programs across

Ohio. In New York, OnTrackNY has more than 20 coordinated specialty care programs across New York City and New York State.

Psychoeducation

As discussed in Chapter 8, **psychoeducation** is a type of education that focuses on the topic of mental illnesses. The goal of psychoeducation is to help individuals with a mental illness, and their family members, better understand the illness. If a person understands his or her illness, then he or she will be able to deal with it more successfully. Psychoeducation, for both young people and their families, is an effective form of treatment in itself and an important step in preventing relapse and hospitalization. Research has shown that those who receive psychoeducation are less likely to have a relapse and be hospitalized compared to those who do not receive psychoeducation.

> The goal of psychoeducation is to help individuals with a mental illness, and their family members, better understand the illness. If a person understands his or her illness, then he or she will be able to deal with it more successfully.

Case Management

Case management is an important part of many programs designed especially for young people with psychosis. Case management is a service in which one person is in charge of checking in with the individual on a regular basis and making sure that he or she has all the services needed. Case managers are usually nurses, social workers, or other health professionals who help young people to coordinate the different parts of their treatment. They can work alone or in teams. Case managers in many programs call or visit the young person at least once a week. They ask how the person is doing and if he or she needs anything. They also help people find and sign up for things like classes, groups, and helpful programs. The purpose is to help someone with psychosis live more independently and to help families as well. The case manager usually talks to the individual's other mental health professionals about any new symptoms or issues that come up. In this way, the case manager helps to make sure that the program is providing the young person with as many helpful treatments and services as possible.

Medicines

Programs for people with a first episode of psychosis always provide an evaluation by a psychiatrist or other medical professional who can prescribe medicines. Most programs for young people with early psychosis start with a low dosage of an antipsychotic medicine (see Chapter 7, "Medicines Used to Treat Psychosis"). The dosage can then be carefully adjusted as needed. Medicines are an important part of the treatment of psychosis.

> In addition to psychoeducation, case management, and antipsychotic medicines, most programs for young people with a first episode of psychosis offer several specific psychosocial treatments. They are called psychosocial treatments because they address both psychological problems (like the symptoms of psychosis) and social problems (like needing to get back to school or work).

Psychosocial Treatments

In addition to psychoeducation, case management, and antipsychotic medicines, most programs for young people with a first episode of psychosis offer several specific **psychosocial treatments**. They are called *psychosocial* treatments because they address both psychological problems (like the symptoms of psychosis) and social problems (like needing to get back to school or work). That is, these treatments aim to help the person with symptoms of psychosis and with other problems that sometimes occur as a result of psychosis. For example, psychosocial treatments may focus on depression, substance use, getting back to school or work, and improving relationships. Psychosocial treatments are very helpful, especially in combination with medicines, for people who are moving toward recovery.

Psychosocial treatments often include individual therapy sessions, classes, or group sessions (see Chapter 8). Cognitive-behavioral therapy, which helps people examine and improve their thoughts and actions, is often the basis for individual therapy sessions. In addition, programs may provide other forms of individual counseling or therapy. Some programs also offer classes on topics such as social skills and employment. These classes help young people to catch up on opportunities that may have been interrupted during the early stages of psychosis, such as learning job skills. This helps young people to get back to school, work, recreational activities, and spending time with friends, which is a part of recovery and leading a fulfilling life. One type of treatment that specifically helps with getting back into school or work is supported education or supported employment.

Community Outreach

Many specialty programs for young people with psychosis provide community outreach to educate people about psychosis and to encourage people to get treatment early. Often, they do two kinds of community outreach at the same time. First, they do general outreach to everyone. The community outreach program may use social media or put posters in public places like bus stations or subway trains. Most programs also have user-friendly websites where the public can find very useful information. Sometimes people who have had psychosis or their family members also take part in helping to educate others about psychosis. The purpose of this kind of public education is to teach everyone about the early symptoms of psychosis, and to help people get treatment earlier.

The second kind of community outreach focuses more on doctors, school counselors, and other people who may meet someone with early psychosis in the community. In these educational programs for doctors, school counselors, and other professionals, the community outreach program sends flyers and may give presentations to make sure they know about the available specialty services. Researchers have found that people come to specialty care programs earlier when there are outreach campaigns in the community. This is important because the earlier evaluation and treatment begins, the better people tend to do in the long term.

Seeking More Information

Your mental health professional (or team) is a great source for more information. Don't be afraid to ask them to explain more, if things are unclear. Another good idea is to bring a list of questions with you when you meet with your mental health professional to make sure that you leave the appointment with all your questions answered. Several worksheets provided in this book—and available in printable form online at www.oup.com/firstepisodepsychosis—can help you keep track of information from your mental health professional, or to share your own experiences and symptoms with your mental health professional. Your treatment program might have similar handouts and other resources. There are a number of very helpful websites that provide more information. Your treatment team will be able to provide written information and recommendations for other books, reliable websites, and more.

Treatments During the Prodromal Phase

In some places, specialized clinics and treatment programs have been developed to try to identify and help young people who may be about to develop psychosis, before the psychosis begins. Such programs do this by providing services to people who appear to be at elevated risk for developing psychosis. These young people have the same types of symptoms seen in the prodromal phase of a psychotic disorder. Usually, before someone has psychosis for the first time, he or she gradually develops milder symptoms, such as social withdrawal, suspiciousness, or unusual ideas. Not everyone who has these types of milder symptoms will go on to develop psychosis, but these symptoms put them at increased risk. For those who do develop psychosis, this period of initial symptoms is called the prodrome, or prodromal phase (see Chapter 1, "What Is Psychosis?").

Treatment programs for people who may be in the prodromal stage can be helpful. They usually consist of psychosocial treatments, similar to the ones listed earlier and explained more thoroughly in Chapter 8. In some cases, psychiatrists in these specialized clinics prescribe a medicine to treat specific symptoms. This can decrease the severity of the symptoms and perhaps even keep the person from having psychosis. However, the psychiatrist will very carefully weigh the benefits and the risks of taking medicine at this early stage and will discuss the benefits and risks with the young person and his or her family. If a medicine is started, the young person will be carefully monitored for the development of any side effects. Also, mental health professionals in these specialized clinics can help people get into specialty treatment as early as possible if they do develop psychosis.

Putting It All Together

If you or someone you know has recently had the onset of psychotic symptoms or has been newly diagnosed with a psychotic disorder, you may find a specialty program for early or first-episode psychosis, like coordinated specialty care, to be particularly helpful. This is because such programs have specially trained mental health professionals and provide the best-proven treatments. In addition to these programs, there are also programs that treat people who appear to be at elevated risk for developing psychosis or who may be in the prodromal phase.

If you are looking for a program, you may be able to find one through an internet search (for example, at https://www.samhsa.gov/esmi-treatment-locator or http://med.stanford.edu/peppnet/interactivedirectory.html) or by asking a mental health professional in your area. If there is no specialty program for early psychosis in your area, you could also look for a treatment facility with mental health professionals who specialize in psychosis or schizophrenia, or a more general program that has some of the same services listed above. If a specialty program is not available, it is still important to find an experienced mental health professional and to create a small team of support who can provide the various components of the services described in this chapter (like medication management, psychoeducation, and psychosocial treatments).

Key Chapter Points

- In many places around the world, there are specialty clinics that are specifically devoted to people with the early stages of psychosis. These are sometimes called early intervention services or coordinated specialty care programs.
- Specialty programs usually do a full evaluation of the young person and provide ongoing medication management as well as a number of psychosocial treatments.
- Many specialty programs for early psychosis also offer classes or group meetings just for young people who have recently been diagnosed with a psychotic disorder, and other group meetings for the families of these young people.
- Specialty programs for early psychosis focus on recovery, shared decision-making, and individuals' life goals. These programs also provide outreach to the community to aid in earlier detection that will hopefully reduce delays to getting into care.
- In some places, specialized clinics and treatment programs have been developed to try to identify and help young people who may be about to develop psychosis, before the psychosis begins. Such programs do this by providing services to people who appear to be at elevated risk for developing psychosis.

6

The Initial Evaluation of Psychosis

Individuals experiencing a first episode of psychosis and their families sometimes hesitate in seeking mental health evaluation and treatment. One reason may be that they don't understand what is happening and they don't know what to expect. In addition, stories from the media, common myths, or other ideas about what happens to people with psychosis may be frightening. But a thorough evaluation is crucial for developing an effective treatment plan. This chapter explains the evaluation provided in a healthcare setting when someone seeks help for a first episode of psychosis.

A thorough evaluation is the first step for mental health professionals to help the person with psychosis. The main reason for evaluation is to better understand what the person is experiencing and to begin planning the best treatment. Early psychosis differs greatly across individuals. It can include many different types of symptoms (see Chapter 2, "What Are the Symptoms of Psychosis?") that are caused by a number of different disorders (see Chapter 3, "What Diagnoses Are Associated with Psychosis?"). A thorough evaluation allows the mental health professional to compile all available information, from different perspectives, to arrive at the most appropriate diagnosis and develop the most effective treatment plan.

As described in Chapter 3, a thorough evaluation assesses three types of possible causes of psychosis:

1. Are the symptoms a result of a medical condition that requires treatment?
2. Are they stemming from drug use?
3. Or do they indicate a psychiatric illness, such as major depression, bipolar disorder, or a primary psychotic disorder such as schizophrenia?

The evaluation process can provide families with an explanation for what their loved one is experiencing. It also may help the person with psychosis to feel better understood. And importantly, it helps them to start on a path toward effective treatment and recovery.

The evaluation process can provide families with an explanation for what their loved one is experiencing. It also may help the person with psychosis to feel better understood. And importantly, it helps them to start on a path toward effective treatment and recovery.

In-depth interviews allow the mental health professional to understand the nature of the psychotic symptoms, including when they started, how they progressed, and what makes them better or worse. In addition to gathering information from the young person experiencing the symptoms, the mental health professional will want to collect any other medical, psychological, or psychiatric records that may be helpful and to possibly also contact others who know the young person to get their perspectives. The mental health professional may refer the young person for medical and/or psychological exams, including a physical exam and lab tests, and perhaps cognitive testing, an electroencephalogram (EEG), and an imaging study, such as a head computerized axial tomography (CAT) scan or magnetic resonance imaging (MRI), which are described later in the chapter.

Before we explain the parts of the evaluation process, it is important to understand the difference between inpatient and outpatient evaluation and treatment settings. Inpatient settings are usually in hospitals, where people stay overnight for several days. The amount of time spent depends on how serious the individual's symptoms are and whether there are any safety concerns. Those receiving services in an outpatient setting visit a mental health professional's office or treatment program for an appointment but then return home. Whether the initial evaluation is done in an inpatient or outpatient setting is usually determined by the mental health professional, the family, and the young person, based on many factors, including how serious the psychotic symptoms are. We return to inpatient versus outpatient settings toward the end of this chapter.

Interviews and Collecting Information

Several different types of mental health professionals may take part in the evaluation process. The initial interview (discussion between the young person experiencing psychosis and the mental health professional) is often done by a psychiatrist or a psychologist. In some places, the initial interview might be done by a social worker, a mental health counselor, or a psychiatric nurse practitioner. A **psychiatrist** is a medical doctor who has received specialty training in psychiatry. Psychiatrists evaluate and treat people with mental illnesses and often prescribe medicines as part of the treatment. A **psychologist** is similar to a psychiatrist but has received training in the field of psychology rather than in medicine. Although psychologists are usually not licensed to prescribe medicines, they have other specialized skills, such as performing formal psychological testing (like the cognitive tests described later in this chapter). Other mental health professionals include social workers, mental health counselors, psychiatric nurse practitioners, psychiatric nurses, case managers, mental health associates, peer specialists, and other trained staff who work as part of the treatment team.

The evaluation process consists of several steps. First, a psychiatrist, psychologist, or another mental health professional will conduct an interview with the young person. This interview helps the mental health professional to understand the difficulties the individual has been experiencing. They will ask many questions to understand these experiences. It is also common for the mental health professional to ask several questions about the young person's family. They will have a number of questions for people who know the young person experiencing psychosis well, like family members. All of these questions help identify specific symptoms that make up the various diagnoses described in Chapter 3. This large amount of information about what has been going on in the past and more recently is sometimes called the *history*. The mental health professional wants to know what symptoms the young person has experienced and the events that led up to the current difficulties. Gathering all of this history includes asking questions about any mental illnesses in family members, previous medical conditions or head injuries, recent social functioning, any recent or past social stressors, any history of trauma, recent or past academic performance, and recent or past substance use.

Mental health professionals sometimes use interview guides to organize their questions when taking the history to better understand the symptoms that the young person is experiencing. When conducting the interview, the mental health professional will often take notes to keep track of everything, and to assist in later putting all the pieces of information together. These notes and the results of all testing described in the following pages become part of the young person's **medical record**. The medical record documents the evaluation and prescribed treatments. It also helps mental health professionals communicate with one another about the person's progress. The medical record is confidential, meaning that only health professionals treating the young person have access to it. The laws defining exactly which health professionals and health agencies have access to it vary across states/provinces and countries. Sometimes the medical record pertaining to the psychosis is separate from the person's physical health medical record, and in other settings they are combined.

In addition to completing a thorough interview, the mental health profession will observe the young person's behavior. Such observations include watching the young person's facial expressions, movements, and body language. Some of the "negative symptoms" cause reduced facial expressions, slowing of movements, or decreased use of gestures, as described in Chapter 2. People who know the individual well, like family members, also may give information about such behaviors and symptoms. Again, family members are very important sources of information during the initial evaluation.

The mental health professional doing the interview will also do a **mental status exam** as part of the interview. The mental status exam includes various questions and observations that assess several aspects of mental functioning, including appearance, attitude, behavior, speech, mood, affect, thought process, thought content, insight, judgment, impulse control, and cognition (Figure 6.1). We will describe each of these so that you understand the types of questions mental health professionals usually ask, and why.

1. *Appearance:* Mental health professionals observe the individual's posture, level of eye contact, and hygiene and grooming. They also look for unusual clothing or hairstyles not typical of the person's cultural background. Sometimes psychotic symptoms like disorganized thinking and disorganized behavior may lead to an odd appearance. Negative symptoms may make it hard for the person to maintain appropriate hygiene.

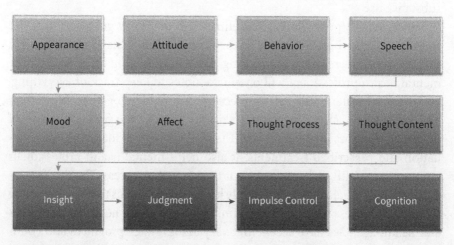

Figure 6.1 Parts of a Mental Status Examination

2. *Attitude:* They also assess the individual's attitude, or the way he or she engages and participates in the interview. Restlessness, anxiety, tension, suspiciousness, and poor cooperation may relate to specific symptoms or disorders.

3. *Behavior:* Mental health professionals look for any odd or unusual behaviors. They also will note any unusual movements, including slowness, tics, tremors, or fidgeting. Negative symptoms may cause a slowing of movements. Some psychotic symptoms may lead to unusual movements, postures, or mannerisms.

4. *Speech:* Mental health professionals also listen carefully to the person's speech. For example, is their speech abnormally slow or fast? Louder or softer than would be expected? Does his or her speech change depending on what he or she is discussing? Or does it lack these normal changes? Does the person give an appropriate response to questions?

5. *Mood:* Mental health professionals also assess the person's mood. For example, is the person happy or sad? They look for mood symptoms such as those that occur with depression or mania.

6. *Affect:* Whereas "mood" is one's own report of one's inner emotional state, "affect" refers to the emotional state as observed by others. Affect is assessed by looking at facial expressions, tone of voice, and gestures. In some cases, the individual will report a mood state that does not match his or her affect. In other cases, the person's affect may appear to be blunted or flat, as described in the discussion of negative symptoms in Chapter 2.

7. *Thought process:* Mental health professionals ask about and observe the person's thought process, which means the ways the thoughts are put together (like the order of thoughts and how each thought is connected to the next). Psychosis sometimes causes disorganization in the thought process, such as tangentiality or loosening of associations. This means that one thought or idea is only loosely associated with the next, such that the thinking is not well connected in a linear and logical way. A person with psychosis may be unaware of disorganized thoughts. However, any disorganization of thinking is often evident to treatment providers and others who have spent time with the individual.

8. *Thought content:* Unlike the thought process, which refers to *how* the person thinks, thought content refers to *what* the person is thinking about. The mental health professional will assess for delusional thoughts, paranoia or suspiciousness, hallucinations, and ideas of reference. Importantly, mental health professionals also almost always ask about

suicidal thoughts and thoughts of harming others. These are standard questions asked of almost all people receiving a mental health evaluation.

9. *Insight:* Insight refers to how well the person understands his or her symptoms and illness. Assessing the level of insight may be helpful in estimating how well the individual will engage in treatment.

10. *Judgment:* Similar to insight, mental health professionals also assess the person's judgment. This can give clues about his or her decision-making ability. Assessing a person's judgment also helps estimate the likelihood of future risky behavior.

11. *Impulse control:* Mental health professionals assess impulse control, or how well a person can stop himself or herself from participating in dangerous behaviors or acting on impulses. Impulse control also explains how well a person thinks through decisions.

12. *Cognition:* The mental status exam also includes a review of the individual's cognitive abilities, including attention, memory, planning skills, and reasoning ability.

The many different questions during the interview and the mental status exam are important to establish a diagnosis and develop a treatment plan. After the interview, history, and mental status exam, mental health professionals may carry out other steps in the evaluation process, described in the following pages. The goal of collecting all of this information during the evaluation is to make treatment recommendations that aim for symptom reduction, improvement in the young person's quality of life, and, ultimately, recovery.

> The goal of collecting all of this information during the evaluation is to make treatment recommendations that aim for symptom reduction, improvement in the young person's quality of life, and, ultimately, recovery.

Other Records and Collateral Information

Sometimes the evaluation may include gathering information from sources other than the young person with psychosis. For example, if the young person has had academic problems, the mental health professional may ask for school records. Similarly, mental health professionals may request medical records from past treatment providers. This is especially important if the young person has had earlier mental health evaluation or treatment.

In many cases, people experiencing psychosis cannot fully explain their recent history because of symptoms such as impaired insight, paranoia, disorganized thoughts, or poor memory. Mental health professionals will try to get **collateral information** from others, such as family members or friends. Collateral information is additional information that may confirm the young person's history or provide another perspective on recent problems. Mental health professionals want this information to get several views on what has been going on.

Physical Exam

Individuals with mental illnesses may have physical illnesses as well. Mental health clinicians often refer individuals with a recent onset of psychosis to a primary care provider for a physical exam to check for medical problems, including those that can cause psychosis, as described in Chapter 3. Individuals receiving services in a hospital or similar inpatient setting often receive a physical exam when admitted to the hospital. The physical exam may include testing eye movements, balance, strength in various muscle groups, and reflexes. The medical doctor will usually also listen to the person's heart and lungs with a stethoscope and may look into their eyes and ears with other instruments. Other parts of the physical exam may rule out the presence of a disease in other parts of the body. In general, the physical exam does not hurt and usually takes about half an hour or less.

Cognitive Tests

Detailed assessments of cognitive functioning are sometimes done, especially in research settings. These assessments can be similar to some of the mental status exam questions described earlier but are even more extensive. Some cognitive functions, like attention, learning, memory, and planning, may be assessed with special verbal or written tests. As noted in Chapter 2 in the discussion of the symptoms of cognitive dysfunction, such tests might include giving the meaning of metaphors, having to follow a series of numbers or letters on a computer screen, having to spell things backward, addition and subtraction, seeing how well things are remembered after several minutes have passed, listing as many animals as possible in a one-minute period, completing a series of mazes, and similar tests. These assessments may identify areas of strengths and weaknesses that are important to consider during treatment planning. Mental health professionals also use these assessments to help in diagnosing some mental illnesses.

Lab Tests

When admitted to the hospital for an episode of psychosis, or even in the outpatient setting, doctors first try to rule out any medical or drug-related causes of psychosis. Drug-induced psychosis might result from drugs like cocaine, ketamine, LSD, marijuana, methamphetamine and other amphetamines, PCP, or synthetic cannabinoids. Doctors use blood and urine tests to check for the presence of drugs and other substances that may cause drug-induced psychosis (also called substance/medication-induced psychotic disorder, as described in Chapter 3). Blood tests may also be ordered to check for infections, vitamin deficiencies, thyroid problems, liver diseases, kidney diseases, and/or neurosyphilis. While it is not common, in some instances, doctors may need to perform a **lumbar puncture** (also called a **spinal tap**) to rule out an infection in the brain by examining cerebrospinal fluid. Such tests may also need to be done to rule out any potential inflammatory process that causes encephalopathy (brain inflammation), which can bring about psychotic symptoms.

Electroencephalogram

Mental health professionals sometimes ask a neurologist to conduct an **electroencephalogram (EEG)** as part of the initial evaluation of psychosis. An EEG records the electrical activity in the brain. To do an EEG, the clinician will attach a number of small electrodes and wires to the person's scalp. The EEG is painless and is commonly used to assess for seizures. Mental health professionals mainly request an EEG to rule out rare seizure disorders, like temporal lobe epilepsy, that sometimes cause psychotic symptoms. Temporal lobe epilepsy is a type of seizure disorder that can mimic a psychotic disorder because it sometimes causes hallucinations or delusions.

Imaging Studies

Although a first episode of psychosis is often due to a psychiatric illness such as a primary psychotic disorder like schizophrenia, **imaging studies** (also called **neuroimaging**) may be done to rule out other causes of psychosis, like a brain tumor. Imaging studies allow radiologists and mental health professionals to look at the brain to determine if there are any abnormal findings, such as a brain tumor or evidence of an infection.

There are several types of imaging studies. One type is a **computerized axial tomography (CAT) scan**, also called a **computerized tomography (CT) scan**, which is similar to a very detailed X-ray of the brain. The X-ray is processed by a computer to produce a picture of the brain. A CT scan mainly looks for brain tumors or other lesions that could cause the psychotic symptoms. A CT scan (rather than one of the other imaging studies described next) is commonly used as part of the initial, or first, evaluation because it is relatively inexpensive. Like the other imaging studies, it is painless, and it is also noninvasive, meaning it does not involve any needles or incisions.

Another type of imaging study is **magnetic resonance imaging** (MRI). An MRI is another noninvasive procedure that shows doctors the brain structure. This allows them to see any abnormalities, such as tumors, swelling inside the brain, or small areas of disease that might cause psychotic symptoms. The MRI uses magnetic waves instead of X-rays.

To have a CT scan or MRI, one must lie down on a bed-like table, which slides into a large tube. When inside an MRI machine, the individual will hear loud noises from the machine. While it is just the machine at work, these sounds do bother some people. Others also might become claustrophobic or fearful of the enclosed space. But these tests do not take long, and they are often important.

If the initial evaluation and treatment are carried out in a clinical research center, researchers may perform other studies as part of an extensive evaluation. This may include specialized imaging studies. A more specialized type of MRI is functional magnetic resonance imaging (fMRI). Other types of research scans include the positron emission tomography (PET) scan and the single photon emission computed tomography (SPECT) scan. These special imaging studies that are used for research measure blood flow in the brain, helping to determine how the brain is functioning. Sometimes, doctors or researchers will ask the person to perform thinking tasks or simple tests during the fMRI or PET scan. Such tasks include things such as remembering or putting items into categories. This helps them determine how different parts of the brain are functioning based on blood flow to those areas.

Combining the Pieces of an Evaluation

The mental health professional uses all of the information gathered from the interview, behavioral observations, mental status exam, other records, collateral information, physical exam, cognitive tests, lab tests, EEG, and imaging studies to make a diagnosis. As discussed in Chapter 3, this sometimes requires an initial working diagnosis and a differential diagnosis until a more certain diagnosis becomes clear. Once all of the information is gathered and the diagnosis is made, the mental health professional will work with the young person and his or her family to help them understand the diagnosis and develop a treatment plan. This treatment plan usually involves a medicine, as discussed in Chapter 7 ("Medicines Used to Treat Psychosis"), as well as one or more psychosocial interventions, described in Chapter 8 ("Psychosocial Treatments for Early Psychosis").

Mental health professionals may be limited in what they can discuss with family members if a young adult has not provided consent for the mental health professional to do so. It is therefore important for individuals receiving services to sign all necessary forms to allow for open communication between the mental health professional and close family members. Confidentiality rules and laws may not allow mental health professionals to share specific information unless consent is given. Such rules generally do not apply to minors as their parents are usually considered their legal guardians and health professionals can share information with them. Additionally, confidentiality rules generally do not apply to life-threatening situations (for example, suicidal thoughts or actions, serious dangerousness, inability to care for self, or during an emergency evaluation) or for general information-sharing (such as education about psychosis in general).

Inpatient Versus Outpatient Evaluation

As mentioned at the beginning of this chapter, mental health professionals conduct evaluations either in an inpatient or an outpatient setting. The level of symptoms and the level of care that is needed largely determine where evaluation and treatment begin. Mental health professionals will recommend hospitalization if the young person poses any possible danger to self or others. They also will recommend hospitalization if the psychosis is serious enough to significantly disrupt the person's functioning or ability to care for himself or herself. In some instances, mental health professionals may be able to initiate treatment in the outpatient setting even if functioning is impaired, as long as there are no immediate safety risks.

Inpatient care (in the hospital or a similar setting) can be either voluntary or involuntary. In the case of **voluntary inpatient treatment**, the young person chooses willingly to sign in to the hospital (or if the young person is a minor, his or her legal guardian [usually a parent] signs them in). On the other hand, **involuntary inpatient treatment** means that the individual has symptoms that require hospitalization, but he or she does not agree to sign in to the hospital. A psychiatrist can then keep the young person in the hospital, depending on state/provincial or national laws. This is also called **involuntary hospitalization, civil commitment,** or **compulsory treatment**. Individuals with severe symptoms that meet specific criteria can be committed from several days to a couple of weeks in most hospital settings. However, commitment can be longer if needed, again depending on state/provincial or national laws. Once acute psychosis lessens, the person will be able to switch from an inpatient to an outpatient treatment setting.

In some areas, **outpatient commitment** (also called **involuntary community treatment** or **assisted outpatient treatment**) may be required when the individual would be best served by outpatient treatment, and a court order is issued to ensure that he or she stays in outpatient treatment. If he or she fails to continue outpatient treatment, then hospitalization may be necessary.

Whether in an inpatient or outpatient setting, mental health professionals encourage young people to be in treatment voluntarily. Voluntary treatment strengthens the working relationship between the young person and his or her mental health professionals, and individuals have better outcomes when voluntarily engaged in treatment.

> Voluntary treatment strengthens the working relationship between the young person and his or her mental health professionals, and individuals have better outcomes when voluntarily engaged in treatment.

Mobile Crisis Teams

Sometimes an initial or follow-up evaluation has to be done at home, especially if the young person refuses to go to see a mental health professional. In some cases, this evaluation might be done by a **mobile crisis team**. These mobile teams usually include two or three people who go to talk with someone who may have psychosis in his or her home, school, or wherever else he or she might be. Mobile teams sometimes also work closely with hotlines. This is so that they can get a phone call from a family member or someone else who is worried about the person. They then try to go and meet with that person who may benefit from an evaluation and referral to treatment.

The mobile team can do an evaluation without always having to take the person to a healthcare setting. They can talk to that person about what is going on and what the options are. If someone is a danger to themselves or others, they may take that person to the hospital for further evaluation and treatment, even if he or she does not want to go. If hospitalization is not necessary, the mobile crisis team makes recommendations and lets the individual and his or her family know about available services.

Sometimes mobile teams work with police officers. Unfortunately, police are sometimes the first people to bring a young person with psychosis in for care. This can be a frightening experience for someone with psychosis. Mobile teams are set up in some cities so that when the police are notified of someone who may have psychosis, a mental health professional can go with an officer to talk to that person and see if he or she needs inpatient or outpatient evaluation and treatment.

Putting It All Together

The evaluation process for psychosis may be unfamiliar or frightening for young people and their family members. There may be many unknowns. While the evaluation process can differ across treatment settings, most evaluations include many parts described in this chapter. These include interviews, reviewing the history, a mental status exam, collecting other records, collateral information, a physical exam, cognitive tests, lab tests, an EEG, and imaging studies. The goal of an evaluation is to better understand what the young person is experiencing, provide an explanation for the young person and the family, give a correct diagnosis, and develop an effective treatment plan that begins the journey toward recovery.

Young people experiencing psychosis, family members, and friends can help the evaluation process by providing important information to mental health professionals, letting mental health professionals know what is most important to them, and seeking information when they are unsure or have questions. Today, many individuals diagnosed with psychosis achieve a meaningful recovery. This would be very unlikely if the individual never came in for an evaluation and treatment. Young people and their family members should not hesitate in seeking treatment. The initial evaluation is the first step toward recovery.

Key Chapter Points

- The evaluation process can provide families with an explanation for what their loved one is experiencing. It also may help the person with psychosis to feel better understood. And importantly, it helps them to start on a path toward effective treatment and recovery.
- Although the initial evaluation can be done in inpatient or outpatient settings, treatment of early psychosis often begins with a short stay in the hospital or related inpatient setting. In some instances, mental health professionals may be able to initiate treatment in the outpatient setting even if functioning is impaired, as long as there are no immediate safety risks.
- Sometimes the evaluation may include gathering additional information from sources other than the young person experiencing psychosis, such as past treatment records.
- Individuals experiencing psychosis often receive a physical exam to look for any medical problems, including medical problems that can cause psychotic symptoms. They also receive lab tests, and possibly other tests.
- Understanding the evaluation process and providing mental health professionals with all available information can help in making a diagnosis and planning for the best treatment that will help the young person move toward recovery.

7

Medicines Used to Treat Psychosis

Mental health professionals treat nearly all psychiatric illnesses using two types of treatments: medicines and psychosocial treatments. This is true for psychosis as well. We describe medicines used to treat psychosis in this chapter and psychosocial treatments for psychosis in Chapter 8, "Psychosocial Treatments for Early Psychosis." Medicines are a crucial part of the treatment plan for people who experience a first episode of psychosis. In fact, psychosocial treatments are usually more effective when medicines help to adequately control symptoms.

We discuss a number of medicines in this chapter. When a specific medicine is mentioned, two names are given. The first is the **generic name** and the second (in parentheses) is the **trade name** in the United States. For example, Tylenol is the trade name of the generic pain medicine called acetaminophen, so we would write that as "acetaminophen (Tylenol)." Anyone taking medicine should be familiar with both the generic and trade names of the medicine, even though the generic names are sometimes more difficult to spell or pronounce.

This chapter begins with an overview of the class of medicines used to treat psychosis, called *antipsychotic medicines*, or just "antipsychotics." Before explaining antipsychotics in further detail, we set the stage by defining (1) how antipsychotics work and (2) some side effects and other serious problems called *adverse events* that may occur when taking antipsychotics. We then describe in more detail the two main types of medicines used to treat psychosis, the *conventional* antipsychotics and the *atypical* antipsychotics. Some mental health professionals refer to these as *first-generation* and *second-generation* antipsychotics, respectively. Then, we discuss the sometimes difficult task of finding the right medicine. We end by addressing two commonly asked questions about antipsychotic medicines: why it's important to take the medicine, and how long it should be taken.

Antipsychotic Medicines

As mentioned earlier, the main types of medicines used to treat psychosis are the **antipsychotics**. These medicines are called *antipsychotics* because they fight against ("anti-") psychotic symptoms. As discussed in Chapters 1 ("What Is Psychosis?") and 2 ("What Are the Symptoms of Psychosis?"), psychosis is when one has hallucinations or delusions. So, the term *antipsychotic medicines* means that this group of medicines works best for positive symptoms such as hallucinations and delusions. Researchers are working to develop medicines that will be helpful for the other types of symptoms associated with psychosis, including negative symptoms and cognitive dysfunction.

> The term *antipsychotic medicines* means that this group of medicines works best for positive symptoms such as hallucinations and delusions. Researchers are working to develop medicines that will be helpful for the other types of symptoms associated with psychosis, including negative symptoms and cognitive dysfunction.

There are over several dozen different antipsychotic medicines in use around the world, giving mental health professionals many options in choosing a medicine to treat hallucinations and delusions. In general, antipsychotic medicines can be divided into two types, the older ones and the newer ones. The older medicines are referred to using various terms, including first-generation antipsychotics, conventional antipsychotics, typical antipsychotics, and neuroleptics. In this chapter, we use the term **conventional antipsychotics** for the older antipsychotics. The newer medicines are referred to either as second-generation antipsychotics or atypical antipsychotics. In this chapter, we use the term **atypical antipsychotics** for the newer medicines.

How Do Antipsychotics Work?

When a person swallows a pill or capsule, some portion of the chemical inside the pill or capsule will be absorbed from the digestive system into the bloodstream. For psychiatric medicines, some portion of this absorbed chemical will then enter the brain from the bloodstream. It is in the brain that antipsychotics have their helpful effects. For the antipsychotics that are available as a long-acting shot usually given every two to four weeks, the chemical in the shot is slowly absorbed from the muscle into the bloodstream and into the brain.

Once in the brain, the active ingredient of the medicine binds to **receptors**. Receptors are proteins on the surface of cells, such as nerve cells, which are also called neurons. When this active ingredient of the medicine binds to the receptor on the surface of a neuron in the brain, the chemical can either "turn on" or "turn off" the receptor (or turn the receptor's activity up some or down some). This binding to the receptor protein therefore either mimics the usual actions of natural chemicals within the brain (turning on or turning up) or decreases the usual actions of such chemicals (turning off or turning down).

This binding and "turning on or turning up" or "turning off or turning down" of the receptor by the medicine then causes further chemical changes that affect the ways that neurons communicate with one another. Nearly all medicines used to treat psychiatric illnesses, including antidepressants, mood stabilizers, anti-anxiety medicines, sleep medicines, and antipsychotics, bind to different types of receptors in brain pathways that regulate mood, anxiety, sleep, thinking, attention, etc.

The one thing the various types of antipsychotics have in common is that they bind to dopamine receptors in the brain. Dopamine is a natural chemical in the brain that allows certain neurons to communicate with one another. Dopamine neurons are involved in movement, pleasure, thinking, and senses such as seeing and hearing. Antipsychotics bind to and turn off or turn down a certain type of dopamine receptor called the D_2 receptor. Doing this turns down the dopamine communication between neurons, which better regulates these brain pathways in individuals with psychosis. The well-known fact that antipsychotic medicines turn down the activity of dopamine receptors on certain neurons has led scientists to think that part of the cause of schizophrenia may be related to abnormal levels of dopamine in certain parts of the brain (see Chapter 4, "What Causes Primary Psychotic Disorders Like Schizophrenia?").

Research has proven that antipsychotic medicines work. In fact, doctors think that all people with psychosis should take an antipsychotic medicine, just as all people with pneumonia due to bacteria should take an antibiotic. That is, they are helpful in decreasing or getting rid of symptoms, such as hallucinations like hearing voices. They are also helpful in decreasing one's focus on delusions, or gradually removing delusions altogether. They treat a number of other symptoms, such as paranoia, as well. They are somewhat helpful for other types of symptoms, though further research is required to develop better medicines to treat negative symptoms and cognitive dysfunction associated with psychosis.

> Research has proven that antipsychotic medicines work. In fact, doctors think that all people with psychosis should take an antipsychotic medicine, just as all people with pneumonia due to bacteria should take an antibiotic.

What Are Side Effects?

Some antipsychotics bind to other types of receptors in the brain, such as **acetylcholine**, **histamine**, **norepinephrine**, and **serotonin** receptors, and this can be the cause of some of the **side effects** of antipsychotics. Side effects are unwanted effects of medicines. For example, an antipsychotic medicine that binds to and turns down acetylcholine receptors in addition to dopamine receptors may cause a dry mouth. Binding to and turning down histamine receptors may lead to drowsiness, and binding to and turning down norepinephrine receptors may lead to changes in blood pressure. Descriptions of side effects that may happen when taking specific antipsychotics follow in the sections "Conventional Antipsychotics" and "Atypical Antipsychotics."

All medicines can cause side effects, but not every person taking a particular medicine will have side effects. In fact, most people do not experience side effects from their medicines. Table 7.1 lists some of the side effects that may occur when taking an antipsychotic medicine. It is important to discuss possible side effects from specific medicines with the psychiatrist or other health professional prescribing the medicine. That way, young people and their families will know which particular ones to look out for and how to handle them if they do occur.

Side effects are most likely to occur when a medicine is just being started, and side effects often go away after several days or weeks of taking the medicine. Mental health professionals are very interested in hearing about whether someone taking medicine is having any side effects. Mental health professionals want to work closely with young people to find the right dose of medicine that works the best, while at the same time minimizing side effects as much as possible.

When a young person has a side effect, the doctor has several options to try to reduce the side effect. Some of these options are as follows:

- If it is likely that the side effect will go away after a few days or weeks, the doctor may ask the individual to try to continue taking the medicine despite having a side effect.

Table 7.1 Common Side Effects That May
Occur When Taking an Antipsychotic Medicine

General side effects	Blurry vision
	Constipation
	Dry mouth
	Headache
	Insomnia (difficulty falling asleep or staying asleep)
	Sexual side effects (such as decreased sex drive)
	Sleepiness/sedation/drowsiness
	Upset stomach (nausea, vomiting, diarrhea)
Secondary negative symptoms	Decreased creativity
	Decreased emotion
	Feeling cloudy or foggy
	Slowness
Extrapyramidal side effects	(see Table 7.3)
Metabolic side effects	(see Table 7.5)
Side effects from elevated prolactin levels	Menstrual irregularities in women
	Breast enlargement, breast tenderness, or milk production in women
	Growth of breast tissue in men
	Weight gain

- The doctor may carefully decrease the dose of the medicine a little to try to get rid of the side effect while keeping the helpful effects.
- The doctor may change the way the young person takes the medicine, such as dividing the dose and taking it twice a day (once in the morning and once at night) instead of once a day.
- The doctor may start another medicine used to treat the side effect.
- The young person may need to switch to another medicine that hopefully will not cause the side effect (see the following pages for ways that doctors switch medicines).

What Are Adverse Events?

Adverse events are similar to side effects in that they are unwanted effects of medicines. As noted earlier, side effects are relatively common, often happen when the young person first starts taking the medicine, and often go away with some time. However, adverse events are more rare, may happen at any time when taking the medicine (not just when starting the medicine or increasing the dose), and sometimes may not go away. Also, whereas side effects are usually mild and often can be tolerated or easily treated, adverse events are serious and at times may even be life-threatening.

Just as all medicines used by doctors to treat any disease can cause some side effects, many medicines can also cause these rare adverse events. Examples of an adverse event are an allergic reaction to penicillin, fainting caused by a blood pressure medicine, swelling of the tongue caused by a blood pressure medicine, bleeding in the stomach caused by a pain medicine, or extremely low blood sugar caused by insulin. These are all serious and require immediate medical attention. Antipsychotic medicines do not cause most of these adverse events, but they can cause other adverse events in rare instances. We describe rare adverse events that may happen when taking specific antipsychotics in later sections of this chapter. When an individual has an adverse event, the doctor often will switch the medicine immediately. Other options may include decreasing the dose, adding another medicine to treat the adverse event, or gradually switching to a different medicine (again, see the following pages for ways that doctors switch medicines).

Conventional Antipsychotics

As mentioned earlier, there are two major types of antipsychotic medicines: conventional antipsychotics (the older ones) and atypical antipsychotics (the newer ones). The conventional antipsychotics were first discovered in the 1950s. Before that time, there were almost no treatments for psychosis in the form of medicines. In the 1950s through the 1980s, a number of conventional antipsychotics were developed. Table 7.2 lists some of these, though there are more than 50 such conventional antipsychotics in use around the world. The conventional antipsychotics are proven to be helpful in reducing the symptoms of psychosis, especially hallucinations, delusions, paranoia, and disorganized thinking. They are less effective—or not effective at all—in treating some of the other types of symptoms, including negative symptoms and cognitive dysfunction.

Some of the side effects that may happen when taking conventional antipsychotics include blurry vision, constipation, dizziness on standing, dry mouth, sleepiness, low blood pressure, and upset stomach. Conventional antipsychotics can also cause a dulling or slowing of thinking and movements

Table 7.2 Some of the Many Conventional
Antipsychotic Medicines Currently Available in the
United States

Generic Name	Trade Name
Chlorpromazine	Thorazine
Fluphenazine	Prolixin
Haloperidol	Haldol
Loxapine	Loxitane
Mesoridazine	Serentil
Molindone	Moban
Perphenazine	Trilafon
Pimozide	Orap
Thioridazine	Mellaril
Thiothixene	Navane
Trifluoperazine	Stelazine

referred to as "secondary negative symptoms" because they mimic the negative symptoms of schizophrenia, but they come from the medicine.

A common set of side effects of conventional antipsychotics are the **extrapyramidal side effects** (EPS, or EPSE). EPS get their name from the extrapyramidal system in the brain, which is a network of neurons that helps to regulate movement in the body. EPS are a number of movement side effects, which we list and define in Table 7.3. EPS can be quite common when taking conventional antipsychotics. They are less likely to occur when taking the newer atypical antipsychotic medicines (described next). Often, EPS are treated by adding another medicine that is used specifically to treat the EPS. Such medicines may include benztropine (Cogentin), diphenhydramine (Benadryl), hydroxyzine (Atarax, Vistaril), or trihexyphenidyl (Artane).

Another side effect that may happen when taking conventional antipsychotics is an elevation in the **prolactin** level in the blood. Prolactin is a hormone secreted by the pituitary gland in the brain. Determining an elevated prolactin level requires drawing a sample of blood to be sent to the lab. An increase in the prolactin level can cause a number of side effects. For example, in women, an increase in the prolactin level can cause breast enlargement or tenderness, and even milk production despite not being pregnant or postpartum. It can also cause the menstrual cycle to become irregular or to stop. In men, an elevated prolactin level can cause the breast tissue to grow. In both men and women, an elevated prolactin level also can be one cause of weight gain. If the prolactin elevation is mild, it may not cause any side

Table 7.3 Various Forms of Extrapyramidal Side Effects (EPS) of Antipsychotic Medicines

Type of EPS	Description	Appearance
Acute dystonia	This side effect usually comes on suddenly, and often when first starting a new medicine. It typically involves painful tightening of a muscle or muscle group.	* Oculogyric crisis: sudden, painful tightening of the eye muscles * Torticollis: sudden, painful neck spasm * Dystonia: the sudden, painful contraction of a muscle or muscle group
Akathisia	An inner sense of restlessness, fidgetiness, or inner need to move. It can occur when first starting a new medicine, or at any time.	* Anxiety * Fidgeting * Pacing * Constant shifting or moving of legs
Parkinsonism	A group of side effects that mimic the symptoms of Parkinson's disease. It can occur when first starting a new medicine, or at any time.	* Decreased facial expression * Fine tremor of the hands * Handwriting becomes very small * Slow, shuffling gait * Slowing of movements * Stiffness of muscles

effects and may not require treatment. However, if the elevation of prolactin level in the blood causes side effects, the doctor will often decrease the dose of the antipsychotic or will add another medicine to reduce the prolactin level. Although an elevated prolactin level is usually an issue only with the conventional antipsychotics, some of the newer atypical antipsychotics described in the following pages, such as risperidone (Risperdal), also may cause elevated prolactin levels.

Several adverse events may happen when taking conventional antipsychotics. Rarely, these medicines can cause an allergic reaction, such as hives and itching, a swollen airway or tongue, or difficulty breathing. In rare instances, conventional antipsychotics can sometimes cause a seizure, especially in people who have a tendency to have seizures or who are taking another medicine that also can increase risk for seizures. Very rarely, such medicines may cause dysfunction of specific organs, like the liver (hepatitis) or the pancreas (pancreatitis).

One important adverse event that is much more common with conventional antipsychotics than with atypical antipsychotics is **tardive dyskinesia (TD)**. TD is an adverse event that develops after extended periods (months, years, or decades) of taking conventional antipsychotics. TD consists of abnormal, involuntary movements. These movements often involve the mouth (chewing or puckering movements), the fingers or toes, or the trunk (such as rocking or swaying). When using conventional antipsychotics, doctors often assess for TD regularly, such as every six months, by carefully observing the tongue, fingers, and toes for abnormal, involuntary movements.

Despite the possibility of producing side effects or adverse events, conventional antipsychotics are very helpful in treating psychosis for many people. In fact, for some people, these older medicines seem to be even more helpful than the newer medicines. However, nowadays most young people with a first episode of psychosis are initially treated with one of the newer medicines, an atypical antipsychotic.

Atypical Antipsychotics

Only conventional antipsychotics were available from the mid- to late 1950s through the early 1990s. Beginning in the 1990s, a newer class of antipsychotics was developed. In addition to binding to and turning off dopamine receptors, these newer medicines also bind to certain **serotonin** receptors. Serotonin is another natural chemical in the brain that appears to play a role in the mental functions affected by psychosis.

You may be wondering why mental health professionals call the newer antipsychotics "atypical." There are several ways in which the newer medicines differ from conventional antipsychotics, leading mental health professionals to call the newer, second-generation antipsychotics "atypical." Some of the reasons for this terminology are:

- The beneficial effects of these medicines appear to be related to the fact that they bind to serotonin receptors in addition to dopamine receptors.
- These medicines may be more helpful in treating certain types of symptoms, like negative symptoms and cognitive dysfunction, compared to the older, conventional medicines, though research has not definitively proven this.
- These medicines are generally less likely to cause EPS.
- Most of these medicines are less likely to cause elevated prolactin levels.
- Perhaps most importantly, these medicines are less likely to cause TD, even after taking them for years.

Like the conventional antipsychotics, atypical antipsychotics have been proven to be helpful in reducing the symptoms of psychosis, especially hallucinations, delusions, paranoia, and disorganized thinking. Some doctors and researchers believe that atypical antipsychotics may be somewhat more effective in treating some of the other types of symptoms, like negative symptoms and cognitive dysfunction, though, as noted earlier, the research support for this is unclear. More than 10 atypical antipsychotics are in use around the world, and many of these are listed, along with the usual daily starting dose and typical effective dose, in Table 7.4.

Many mental health professionals view atypical antipsychotics as the first-choice medicines for the treatment of psychosis. So, doctors often prefer to use these newer medicines first, reserving the older medicines for use only if atypical antipsychotics prove unsuccessful. Unfortunately, the atypical antipsychotics can be more expensive than the conventional antipsychotics.

Researchers have studied the effects of atypical antipsychotics on other psychiatric illnesses, in addition to psychosis. Government agencies (like the Food and Drug Administration [FDA] in the United States) have approved some of these medicines for the treatment of bipolar disorder, major depression, and other disorders in addition to psychosis.

Some of the side effects that may happen when taking atypical antipsychotics include the same side effects that may occur when taking conventional antipsychotics: blurry vision, constipation, dizziness on standing, dry mouth, sleepiness, low blood pressure, and upset stomach. As noted earlier, most atypical antipsychotics are less likely to cause EPS and elevated prolactin levels. In general, atypical antipsychotics are usually well tolerated,

Table 7.4 Atypical Antipsychotic Medicines Currently Available in the United States

Generic Name (Trade Name)	Usual Daily Starting Dose	Typical Daily Effective Dose
Clozapine (Clozaril)	25 mg	400–600 mg
Risperidone (Risperdal)	1–2 mg	2–6 mg
Olanzapine (Zyprexa)	5–10 mg	10–30 mg
Quetiapine (Seroquel)	100–200 mg	300–800 mg
Ziprasidone (Geodon)	40–80 mg	120–240 mg
Aripiprazole (Abilify)	5–15 mg	10–30 mg
Paliperidone (Invega)	3–6 mg	3–12 mg
Iloperidone (Fanapt)	1–2 mg	6–24 mg
Lurasidone (Latuda)	20–40 mg	40–80 mg
Asenapine (Saphris)	5–10 mg	10–20 mg
Brexpiprazole (Rexulti)	1 mg	2–4 mg

meaning that they usually do not cause many side effects. This is especially true when these medicines are used at relatively low doses, which is often the case for individuals going through the initial evaluation and treatment of a first episode of psychosis.

Two important types of side effects that can occur when taking some of the atypical antipsychotics (and also many of the conventional antipsychotics) are **weight gain** and **metabolic side effects**. These side effects are especially likely to occur with clozapine (Clozaril) and olanzapine (Zyprexa), but nearly any antipsychotic medicine may stimulate appetite and cause weight gain. Because of the possibility of these side effects, doctors prescribing atypical antipsychotics closely monitor the person's weight and periodically check certain labs, like **fasting glucose and lipids** (lipids include triglycerides and cholesterol) (Table 7.5). This requires drawing a sample of blood to be sent to the lab. Careful monitoring for weight gain and metabolic side effects is crucial because both have negative long-term health consequences. If the doctor sees that such side effects are developing, he or she may try one or more of the strategies listed earlier to get rid of the side effects.

One of the atypical antipsychotics, called clozapine (Clozaril), has unparalleled effectiveness for positive symptoms (hallucinations and delusions), especially if other antipsychotic medicines have not worked. Unfortunately, clozapine can cause several adverse events, including serious (and even life-threatening) constipation, agranulocytosis (a sudden and dangerous drop in the white blood cell count that leaves the person susceptible to severe infections), myocarditis (an inflammation of the heart muscle), and seizures. Though rare, because of the risk of agranulocytosis, those taking clozapine must have weekly (or biweekly) blood draws to closely monitor the white blood cell count. That is, those taking clozapine in the United States (with similar protocols in other countries) must have weekly blood draws for the first six months, every other week from month six to 12, and then monthly

Table 7.5 Weight Gain and Metabolic Side Effects That May Be Caused by Atypical Antipsychotic Medicines and Ways Doctors Monitor for These Side Effects

Side Effects	Ways to Monitor
Weight gain	Waist circumference, body weight, body mass index
Metabolic side effects * Elevated triglycerides * Elevated cholesterol * Elevated glucose (sugar)	Blood samples for fasting lipids (triglycerides and cholesterol) and fasting glucose

after one year. This is necessary even though the risk of agranulocytosis is only about 1%. Constipation is also carefully monitored for, and other medicines are often given to prevent serious constipation.

The risk of these adverse events with clozapine is particularly unfortunate because, of all of the antipsychotics, clozapine is the one that is most helpful in treating psychosis that does not respond to other antipsychotics. In fact, clozapine is often reserved for individuals with **treatment-resistant psychosis**, meaning that the psychotic symptoms have not cleared up even after trying two or more different antipsychotic medicines. Clozapine is more helpful than other medicines for treatment-refractory psychosis.

Finding the Right Antipsychotic Medicine

Research shows that atypical antipsychotics may be somewhat more effective than conventional antipsychotics. This is because they may treat a wider range of symptoms, though this is not always the case. However, all of the atypical antipsychotics appear to be about equally effective (except for the fact that clozapine is more effective than other medicines when psychosis continues despite using other medicines). So, doctors select from among the various antipsychotic medicines based on a number of other factors. These may include:

- whether or not the medicine helped in the past
- the specific symptoms present
- past side effects or expected side effects (for example, if someone hasn't been sleeping well, and a particular medicine can also help with sleep)
- how easy it is to take the medicine (for example, once rather than twice daily)
- the cost of the medicine
- the doctor's own familiarity with specific medicines
- whether or not a family member ever benefited from the medicine

Doctors usually consider all of these factors when working with the young person with psychosis and his or her family to select a medicine. The doctor tries to maximize the benefits in terms of symptom response, while minimizing side effects and adverse events.

Sometimes the first medicine that is tried is successful. Other times, the first medicine may cause side effects or may not work. In these cases, the doctor may need to switch to another medicine. Usually after one to three different medicines are tried, the best medicine can be identified. In other cases, if psychotic symptoms are severe, the doctor may want to try a higher dose or increase the dose more rapidly.

Doctors usually try to find the lowest effective dose in order to minimize side effects. This is called *low-dose medication management* and is the recommended framework for prescribing medicines to young people with first-episode psychosis. The symptoms of first-episode psychosis often clear up fairly well with a relatively low dose of the antipsychotic. Individuals with a first episode of psychosis also may be more likely to develop side effects than older individuals who have been taking medicines longer. For these reasons, doctors often try to find the lowest does that is still effective. However, a dose that is too low may not provide all of the benefits that could be seen with a higher dose. So, doctors work to find a "therapeutic dose" without using more medicine than is necessary.

If the doctor recommends that the medicine be switched to another one (perhaps because of side effects or because of inadequate response), the doctor will decide among several ways for how the switch can be done. The switch must be done carefully because any time an antipsychotic medicine is being stopped there is a risk for a relapse of psychotic symptoms. Three methods for making a switch to another medicine are:

- The doctor may stop the first medicine and start the second one.
- The doctor may gradually decrease, or "taper," the first medicine while the second one is being increased, or "titrated," over several days or weeks.
- The doctor may add and increase the second medicine over several days or weeks until it is at an effective dose and then taper or stop the first medicine.

Some young people have a hard time consistently taking their medicine. For these individuals, or for those who would rather simply take a shot than a daily pill, several antipsychotic medicines are available as a shot that is given usually every two to four weeks. Specifically, several conventional antipsychotics are available as a shot, including haloperidol (Haldol) decanoate and fluphenazine (Prolixin) decanoate. A number of atypical antipsychotics, including risperidone, paliperidone, and aripiprazole, are also available as a shot. These injectable medicines ensure that a steady dose of the drug is delivered to the brain while avoiding the inconvenience of having to take pills once or twice a day.

Several atypical antipsychotics are also available as a special rapidly dissolving tablet, in addition to the regular types of pills or capsules. These special tablets dissolve rapidly (within seconds) when placed in the mouth. With these, the young person does not have to swallow a pill. Medicines are now also being developed in a patch form that can be placed on the skin.

Other Medicines Sometimes Used in the Treatment of Psychotic Disorders

Sometimes it is necessary to use other types of medicines, in addition to antipsychotics, to target other types of symptoms. For example, **antidepressants** may be helpful if symptoms of depression are present. **Mood stabilizers** may be useful if irritability, impulsiveness, hostility, or unstable moods are part of the illness. **Anxiety medicines** or **sleep medicines** may be needed if anxiety symptoms or difficulty sleeping is a problem. As mentioned earlier, sometimes medicines used to treat the side effects of antipsychotics, like constipation or EPS, for example, may be needed to make it easier to take the antipsychotic medicine. Nearly all of these other medicines are given as a pill or capsule taken orally. Like any other medicine, these medicines also may cause some side effects in some people.

Possible Future Treatments for Psychotic Disorders

Many researchers around the world are working to discover new medicines that will be even more helpful in treating psychosis. Some of the new medicines that will become available in the upcoming years may be very different from the conventional antipsychotics and the atypical antipsychotics. They might work in different ways, beyond binding to dopamine or serotonin receptors. Additionally, they will hopefully treat a broader range of the symptoms of psychosis. Whereas currently available antipsychotic medicines mainly treat the positive symptoms (like hallucinations and delusions), medicines being developed also will hopefully treat negative symptoms and cognitive dysfunction. This is very important research because, as discussed in Chapter 2, negative symptoms and cognitive dysfunction lead to a lot of the disability associated with schizophrenia and other psychotic disorders.

Why Is It Important to Take the Medicine?

Extensive scientific research has proven that antipsychotic medicines, both conventional and atypical antipsychotics, are effective in reducing the symptoms of psychosis. They are especially helpful in decreasing the positive symptoms, such as auditory hallucinations, delusions, paranoia, and ideas of reference. They are also helpful for disorganized thinking. Antipsychotics may help to some extent with negative symptoms and cognitive dysfunction. As noted in the prior paragraph, ongoing research aims to find even better medicines for psychosis, especially medicines that will be more helpful for negative symptoms and cognitive dysfunction.

Also as noted earlier, many doctors would say that antipsychotic medicines are the most important first step in the treatment of psychosis. By improving the symptoms, young people are better able to benefit from psychosocial treatments (see Chapter 8) designed to promote recovery (see Chapter 12, "Embracing Recovery"). It is very important that individuals with psychosis take their medicines regularly, exactly as prescribed. Sticking with the treatment plan is essential to getting better (see Chapter 9, "Follow-Up and Sticking with Treatment").

The benefits of taking antipsychotic medicines can be thought of in terms of short-term benefits and long-term benefits. The main short-term benefit is the reduction in psychotic symptoms. The long-term benefits of taking antipsychotic medicines stem from this reduction in psychotic symptoms. That is, symptoms are much more likely to clear up when taking antipsychotic medicines, and importantly, the reduction in psychotic symptoms allows one to more easily reach personal goals in areas such as school, work, relationships, and recreation/leisure. In addition to reducing symptoms and promoting recovery, another long-term benefit of taking antipsychotic medicines is that they reduce the chances of a relapse of psychotic symptoms or hospitalization (Figure 7.1). So, in addition to treating psychotic symptoms in the present, antipsychotic medicines have an important role in relapse prevention for the future.

> In addition to reducing symptoms and promoting recovery, another long-term benefit of taking antipsychotic medicines is that they reduce the chances of a relapse of psychotic symptoms or hospitalization. So, in addition to treating psychotic symptoms in the present, antipsychotic medicines have an important role in relapse prevention for the future.

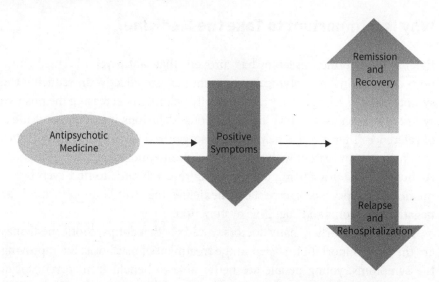

Figure 7.1 The Short-Term and Long-Term Benefits of Antipsychotic Medicines

For How Long Should the Medicine Be Taken?

The first step in the process of taking an antipsychotic medicine is the initial stabilization. Here, the goal is to get rid of the positive symptoms (this is sometimes called **remission**). Approximately 85% of young people with new-onset or first-episode psychosis are able to achieve symptom remission over the course of about three months or so. In many cases, remission may occur even sooner. In general, hallucinations, like hearing voices, may get much better or go away after several days to several weeks on the medicine. Delusions and disorganized thinking may take longer, often several weeks to several months, to get better or go away. This is another reason why it is crucial to stay on the medicine—so that the full effects can be seen over time.

Doctors want to work closely with young people with psychosis to decide how long they should take medicines. In some cases, it is clear to the doctor, based on the types of symptoms present, that the medicine should be continued long term, perhaps even lifelong. In other cases, if symptoms seem to resolve completely, the doctor may recommend a very gradual and careful reduction of the dose. This would usually only happen after complete remission of symptoms for at least six months.

Some young people with psychosis eventually may be able to stop taking the medicine. This is done very carefully with the person and his or her mental health professionals working closely together. Instead of stopping suddenly, the medicine may be gradually decreased over several months. Young people, their families, and their mental health professionals must watch for any return of symptoms or early warning signs (see Chapter 10). However, most who have had an episode of psychosis and receive a diagnosis of a psychotic disorder like schizophrenia will need to continue the medicine long term.

People who experience a first episode of psychosis should not stop their medicines suddenly and should not decrease or stop their medicines without working closely with their doctor. Any change in the dose of the medicine needs very close monitoring. Sometimes this close monitoring may require drawing a blood sample to check the level of the medicine in the bloodstream. This may help the doctor to decide if the dose is right. Fortunately, antipsychotic medicines are not addictive or habit-forming.

Recent research suggests that one of the biggest challenges in the treatment of psychosis is that many young people stop their medicine on their own. For example, some studies show that approximately 70% of those being treated in the early course of a psychotic disorder stop taking the medicine within one year. Common reasons for stopping the medicine may be because it is not working well enough, because of side effects, or because the young person simply decides to stop taking it for other reasons. Some people stop taking medications after they feel better and are not noticing symptoms, but it is important to remember that antipsychotic medicines can play an important role in both treating current symptoms and preventing a return of symptoms in the future. Also, substance use can interfere with the young person's ability to continue taking the medicine as prescribed. Stopping the medicine is problematic because it greatly increases the chance of relapse of symptoms, sometimes requiring hospitalization. Furthermore, stopping the medicine commonly interferes with a person's ability to continue pursuing his or her goals for recovery. For these reasons, mental health professionals usually strongly encourage individuals with a psychotic disorder to take the medicine exactly as prescribed. If the young person does stop taking the medicine, the doctor will want to continue seeing him or her and providing support in other ways, such as counseling and psychoeducation. Worksheet 7.1 can be helpful for keeping track of medicines and changes in medicines. It is also available in printable form at www.oup.com/firstepisodepsychosis.

Putting It All Together

Both conventional and atypical antipsychotic medicines are helpful in reducing psychotic symptoms. These medicines work by blocking and therefore "turning off or turning down" certain types of receptors on neurons in the brain, such as dopamine and serotonin receptors. Side effects may occur with any medicine, including antipsychotic medicines. Different antipsychotic medicines have different types of possible side effects and adverse events. For example, whereas conventional antipsychotics can cause extrapyramidal side effects (EPS), elevated prolactin levels, or tardive dyskinesia (TD), the newer atypical antipsychotics may cause weight gain and metabolic side effects in some people.

Because antipsychotics are proven to be effective in reducing psychotic symptoms, and because side effects may happen, doctors work closely with individuals with psychosis and their families to balance the benefits and risks and find the right medicine and right dose for each person with psychosis. Mental health professionals recommend that the medicine be continued as prescribed to improve one's likelihood of remission. This in turn provides longer-term benefits by promoting recovery and preventing relapse.

Worksheet 7.1 Medicines Prescribed

The amount of information that you have to keep track of can be overwhelming at times. Here is a place to write down your prescribed medicines. It also is a place to keep instructions for taking those medicines.

1. Name of Medicine	Dose

When and How Often to Take the Medicine	Special Instructions from Doctor

2. Name of Medicine	Dose

When and How Often to Take the Medicine	Special Instructions from Doctor

3. Name of Medicine	Dose

When and How Often to Take the Medicine	Special Instructions from Doctor

Key Chapter Points

- Many mental health professionals view medicines to be the most important aspect of the treatment of psychosis.
- The main types of medicines used to treat psychosis are antipsychotics, which are most effective for positive symptoms like hallucinations and delusions.
- Antipsychotics work by binding to dopamine (and, in some cases, serotonin) receptors in the brain, which affects the ways neurons communicate with each other.
- There are two types of antipsychotics: conventional antipsychotics (the older ones) and atypical antipsychotics (the newer ones).
- Sometimes antipsychotics cause side effects. It is important to discuss possible side effects from specific medicines with the psychiatrist, so that individuals with psychosis and their families know which side effects to expect and how to handle them if they happen.
- Low-dose medication management is recommended for young people with first-episode psychosis. Doctors usually try to find the lowest effective dose in order to minimize side effects.
- The length of time that the medicine should be taken is based on the types of symptoms one experiences and how long the symptoms last.

8
Psychosocial Treatments for Early Psychosis

People experiencing psychosis often have to deal with a number of challenges. These challenges may stem from certain symptoms. As explained in Chapter 2 ("What Are the Symptoms of Psychosis?"), these symptoms may include hearing voices or having unusual beliefs; being isolated, withdrawn, or slowed down; and having difficulties with attention, learning, or memory. However, difficulties with school, work, relationships, and recreation/leisure activities may disrupt life as well, and often stem from the experience of psychosis. Young people experiencing psychosis often face these types of challenges. Addressing these difficulties in addition to the specific symptoms is necessary to begin to feel better and to live a full life. In fact, the recovery process focuses as much on resuming school, work, relationships, and recreation/leisure activities as it does on treating symptoms (see Chapter 12, "Embracing Recovery"). Although medicines are extremely important in treating symptoms (see Chapter 7, "Medicines Used to Treat Psychosis"), other types of treatments, called *psychosocial treatments*, focus more on helping young people with these broader areas of difficulty so that they can achieve personal goals.

Psychosocial Difficulties Caused by Psychosis

Psychosocial development begins in childhood and continues throughout adolescence and early adulthood. Adolescence and early adulthood are very important times when people develop social skills and build relationships. This period is typically a time of finishing high school, starting college, getting a first job, having a first romantic relationship, beginning to live more independently from one's parents, getting one's first car, and establishing career goals. Success in all of these life domains requires both psychological skills and social skills. The term *psychosocial* brings together these two words. So, psychosocial development refers to the important developmental stage when psychological and social skills mature.

Late adolescence and early adulthood is also the period of time when a first episode of psychosis usually begins. Thus, psychosis that first happens during this time period often interrupts psychosocial development. Some difficulties that are common among young people experiencing an episode of psychosis include the following:

- declining grades
- dropping out of school
- difficulty getting along with coworkers
- losing a job
- not having friends
- conflicts within the family
- conflicts within a relationship
- trouble maintaining housing
- not maintaining personal hygiene
- giving up hobbies
- having no recreation/leisure activities
- smoking or alcohol/drug use
- not taking care of physical health and well-being

Psychosocial Treatments

As described earlier, individuals experiencing a psychotic episode in late adolescence or early adulthood typically face an interruption in psychosocial development. The goal of psychosocial treatments is to help young people with psychosis or other serious mental illnesses overcome psychological and social challenges and resume a full life. Mental health professionals sometimes use the term **psychosocial rehabilitation** to describe many psychosocial treatments. This means that treatment improves psychosocial skills so that individuals can function in their lives at the best possible level. In other words, psychosocial rehabilitation aims to reduce the challenges young people experience and to maximize abilities in areas such as school, work, relationships, and recreation/leisure.

> The goal of psychosocial treatments is to help young people with psychosis or other serious mental illnesses overcome psychological and social challenges and resume a full life.

There are several types of psychosocial treatments. In some cases, mental health professionals recommend several different treatments at once. These treatments are almost always given in combination with a medicine to treat key symptoms. Just as medicines can improve success in psychosocial treatments, psychosocial treatments (like cognitive-behavioral therapy, psychoeducation, and family psychoeducation) can improve a young person's success with medicine. While the main purpose of medicine is to lessen the severity of symptoms such as hallucinations, psychosocial treatments can focus on symptoms as well as on other areas of life affected by psychosis, like school and work success, relationships, and quality of life. In this way, medicine and psychosocial treatments complement each other as they can target the same and different aspects of the illness.

Although having a decrease in symptoms may make psychosocial treatments easier, it is not necessary for psychosocial interventions. For example, in cognitive-behavioral therapy (described later in this chapter), the basis for a successful therapy is often good rapport (a good working relationship with the therapist), which then allows in-depth discussions to occur about the individual's beliefs about themselves and their environment. This then facilitates the identification of effective strategies that the person can use to develop a more flexible way of understanding their experiences and work on ways to achieve personal goals. This process usually creates opportunities for delusions or hallucinations to begin to shift. Finding a trusted mental health professional and treatment that is person-centered and focused on individual goals is the most important starting point.

Starting and Sticking with Psychosocial Treatments

Many young people and their families are scared to begin treatment because they do not know what to expect. However, getting help as early as possible will lead to the best results. After an initial thorough evaluation (see Chapter 6, "The Initial Evaluation of Psychosis"), the mental health professional may recommend one or more psychosocial treatments in addition to medicine. If the mental health professional doing the initial evaluation is not able to provide the treatments, he or she may give a referral to another professional or program. A **referral** is when a healthcare professional recommends that a person goes to a particular type of treatment.

The time in psychosocial treatments depends on individual need and the type of treatment. For example, residential programs where people live (such as supportive housing), assertive community treatment (described later in the chapter), or day treatment programs may be longer term. We discuss the importance of sticking with treatment in Chapter 9, "Follow-Up and Sticking with Treatment."

A number of different psychosocial treatments are useful for many different mental illnesses, not just psychosis. Psychosocial treatments may be available in several treatment settings, including hospitals, mental health clinics, and private offices of mental health professionals. Some are available in programs that focus specifically on young people with a first episode of psychosis. We discuss these specialized programs in Chapter 5, "Finding the Best Care."

Psychosocial treatment plans may consist of a single psychosocial treatment. But in some cases, combining several psychosocial treatments may be more effective because they allow young people and their families to begin working on several types of challenges at once. We describe 10 different types of psychosocial treatments in the following pages and summarize them in Table 8.1.

Cognitive-Behavioral Therapy

One type of counseling sometimes used for people experiencing psychosis is **cognitive-behavioral therapy** (CBT). CBT targets the specific thoughts and beliefs that an individual has that interfere with life. It assumes that one's thoughts affect both feelings and behaviors and vice versa.

What does this mean that one's "thoughts affect both feelings and behaviors"? Here's an example. A teenaged boy named Aaron was not picked for the school football team and felt bad. Therefore, he then did not want to talk to his friend Tim, who had been picked for the team. A CBT approach may help Aaron start identifying some of the thoughts he experienced when he was not picked, such as "I am a loser." Aaron then is taught to start paying attention to the connection between his thoughts and his feelings. For example, his thought that he is a loser then made him feel sad. If he would have had a different thought under the same circumstances, such as "It's great that I didn't get picked because I can focus more on some things other than football," then he might not have felt sad under the same circumstances. In CBT, the therapist would also help Aaron understand the connection between his thoughts, feelings, and behaviors in specific circumstances. For example, Aaron also had the thought that he must be a worse player than his friend Tim, and so he did not speak to Tim when he saw him. Thus, Aaron's thought (that he was a "loser"), which may not have been completely accurate, affected

Table 8.1 Types of Psychosocial Interventions and Care Delivery Models

Type	Description
Cognitive-Behavioral Therapy (CBT)	Targets specific thoughts and beliefs that make symptoms worse. Often consists of weekly sessions, each lasting 30–60 minutes, led by a counselor specializing in this type of therapy for at least 16 visits over at least six months.
Group Therapy	A discussion or planned activity with a group of individuals led by one or two mental health professionals. Can either be learning about psychosis in a structured way (psychoeducational groups), exploring stressors, relationships, and coping styles (therapy groups), or based on structured activities (activity groups).
Family Interventions	Helps families to cope with stress, improve their social supports, and reduce the effects of stigma. Interventions range from teaching family members about early psychosis and things to expect (family psychoeducation, multi-family groups) to improving communication and problem-solving skills among members (family therapy, Open Dialogue).
Cognitive Remediation	Aims to improve cognitive performance, including difficulties with attention, learning, memory, and planning through individual sessions or in groups. Computer programs or games are often used for practice.
Supported Employment and Supported Education	Helps individuals with psychosis find and keep jobs, as well as achieve educational goals. Provides services including vocational and educational counseling; assessment of skills, abilities, and interests; support services; and job placement assistance.
Social Skills Training	Helps individuals to improve or regain their prior level of social skills, or to resume development of social skills. May be given as a single group session, as an ongoing weekly treatment, or as a part of other psychosocial treatments.
Substance Use Treatment Programs	Programs aimed to target substance use problems for individuals who have a co-occurring disorder. Examples of programs include 12-step programs and integrated dual-diagnosis treatment programs.
Day Treatment and Partial Hospitalization Programs	Outpatient centers that provide treatment daily during working hours. Often serve as a "step-down" after an inpatient hospitalization. Differ in types of treatment offered, but many offer psychosocial interventions in addition to life skills training
Assertive Community Treatment (ACT)	Brings treatment opportunities to individuals in their own settings. Typically, there is no time limit on services, but unfortunately ACT programs are not available in all communities.
Supportive Housing	Provides people with serious mental illnesses a place to live that is supportive and understanding. Housing options could include a private apartment, an apartment shared with a roommate, or a group home.

his feelings (causing him to feel sad), and both his thoughts and his feelings affected his behaviors (causing him to avoid talking to his friend Tim). CBT would teach Aaron to evaluate his thoughts in a more balanced way so that he does not feel sad and avoid Tim. CBT might also teach Aaron to change his behaviors (for example, encourage him to talk with Tim) because this positive interaction might help him feel better and therefore stop thinking that he is a loser.

CBT is a commonly used form of psychotherapy that is helpful for a variety of mental illnesses, including depression, anxiety, and eating disorders. In the case of depression, CBT may help young people to stop thinking of negative things that make them feel down and depressed or start engaging in behaviors that help them feel better and in turn change their negative thoughts. For individuals with psychosis, CBT helps them to consider other explanations for symptoms like delusional ideas, paranoia, and hearing voices, and to develop effective strategies for managing these experiences.

The therapist encourages the individual to pay attention to the various pieces of information available in their environment that provide evidence for and against their beliefs about what is happening. The young person learns to do behavioral experiments to evaluate this information and figure out how it fits into their belief system and then develop a more balanced interpretation of what is happening. The person then practices different strategies and behaviors to cope with the situation and, therefore, feel better.

A similar approach is taught for understanding and managing auditory hallucinations, which helps the person develop a more balanced explanation of what is happening (for example, the voices are not controlling me) and find effective strategies for managing the experience. Through CBT, the young person can also learn helpful coping strategies, such as distraction and relaxation, to improve how he or she feels and relate to others. CBT may also be helpful in targeting and improving negative symptoms partly by finding ways to encourage individuals to become more active and involved in activities that they find important. The overall goal in CBT is to help the person move forward with the things they value and want to accomplish in their lives.

> The overall goal in CBT is to help the person move forward with the things they value and want to accomplish in their lives.

CBT often consists of weekly sessions, each lasting 30 to 60 minutes, led by a counselor specializing in this type of therapy. Often, CBT for psychosis lasts for at least 16 visits over at least six months and may require booster sessions. After therapy ends, young people often continue to use the skills learned in

CBT to manage their symptoms. CBT can also help young people with psychosis to identify early signs of a relapse. Recognizing early warning signs helps them act quickly at the earliest sign of a return of psychotic symptoms (see Chapter 10, "Knowing Your Early Warning Signs and Preventing a Relapse").

In addition to CBT, some young people with psychosis may benefit from other forms of individual therapy or counseling. One example is **supportive psychotherapy**, which supports and builds one's best coping skills. Another example is **acceptance and commitment therapy**, which uses acceptance and mindfulness strategies that encourage one to open up to unpleasant feelings, to learn how to not overreact to them, and to not avoid situations where such feelings might come up.

Group Therapy

While individual psychotherapy, such as CBT, usually takes place one on one between the young person and a mental health professional, **group therapy** is when one or two mental health professionals lead a group of young people in a discussion or a planned activity. Group therapy may be available in an inpatient (hospital) or outpatient (clinic) treatment setting. Group therapy allows young people to learn not only from the therapist, but also from the interactions between the therapist and other group members, and the interactions between group members themselves. This form of psychosocial treatment also can help young people to feel less alone by showing them that others are going through similar difficulties and how they are coping. Group therapy often takes one of three forms: psychoeducational groups, therapy groups, or activity groups.

> Group therapy allows young people to learn not only from the therapist, but also from the interactions between the therapist and other group members, and the interactions between group members themselves. This form of psychosocial treatment also can help young people to feel less alone by showing them that others are going through similar difficulties and how they are coping.

Psychoeducational groups are helpful because they teach young people about psychosis in a clear, structured way, similar to a small class. In psychoeducational groups, young people learn from mental health professionals about symptoms, treatments, early warning signs, and other topics relevant to psychosis.

Therapy groups focus more on helping young people explore their relationships, their coping styles, and stressors that may make symptoms worse. Young people work on understanding themselves and the things they do that may interfere with psychosocial success.

Activity groups are based on structured activities. Thus, the focus is less on learning or counseling and more on experiences and activities. These groups work on developing social skills, confidence, and in some cases job-related skills.

Family Interventions

Families of young people in the early stages of psychosis often experience significant stress from trying to help their loved one manage the illness and navigate the mental health system. Family members or other caregivers may lack social support while caring for an ill family member or may be concerned about the effects of the stigma associated with psychosis. Family interventions help families to cope with stress, improve their social supports, and reduce the effects of stigma. They also often focus on building skills around problem-solving and communication. While we briefly review family interventions provided by mental health professionals here, Chapter 14 ("Reducing Stress, Coping, and Communicating Effectively") focuses on what young people with psychosis and their families can do to strengthen the family during this stressful time. Although we use the term "family," this is a broad term that includes anyone the young person identifies as part of his or her support system, biological or otherwise.

There are several forms of **family interventions**, all of which focus on helping the family as a whole rather than just the young person. Such interventions view each member of the family as having an important role or purpose. Without that member's involvement in the family system, the system would not work as well. Family interventions help both the young person and his or her family by involving each available member of the family. When one member of the family becomes ill from a physical or mental illness, other family members experience some level of distress and everyone's lives become disrupted. In the same way, stress within the family often greatly affects the person with the illness. Family interventions can be divided into family psychoeducation and family therapy, though in many instances these occur within the same family intervention.

Family psychoeducation educates family members about early psychosis and the types of experiences that they can expect when a loved one has psychosis. Like individual psychoeducation or psychoeducational groups for young people with psychosis themselves, family psychoeducation teaches family members about symptoms, diagnoses, evaluations, treatments, and other topics relevant to psychosis. Additionally, and perhaps most importantly, family members learn to recognize the symptoms of a relapse (early warning signs). They also learn strategies for reducing the chance of future relapses. Family psychoeducation may take place in several sessions over an extended period of time, sometimes with weekly or monthly meetings lasting 30 to 90 minutes. The series of sessions may last for several weeks or months.

Led by a mental health professional, family psychoeducation may take place within a single family or within multi-family groups, in which family members from several different families that are going through the same thing are present. Multi-family groups can be helpful because family members can talk to and learn from other families who also have a loved one experiencing psychosis. The young person may or may not be present when family psychoeducation takes place in multi-family groups.

Family therapy is another form of family intervention that may be helpful in reducing the chance of relapse or rehospitalization after a first episode. This is because family therapy directly targets stressors in the young person's immediate environment. Research has shown that family stress may worsen the symptoms of someone in the early stages of psychosis, possibly leading to a relapse. Family therapy focuses on improving communication and problem-solving skills. It strengthens the family's best coping skills, while minimizing challenges and interaction styles that could create stress.

Open Dialogue is an approach to treatment that was first developed in Finland and is now being used in some areas of the United States and other countries. Research is currently being done to look at whether this model could be an effective approach for young people experiencing a first episode of psychosis. The model is a person-centered approach that builds on the strengths of the individual at the center of concern and promotes shared decision-making. It can be used to help people plan their treatment, or what to do if they are in crisis, or to support an individual and their family in an ongoing way. Open Dialogue treatment is carried out through network meetings involving the young person, his or her family members and social network, and at least two mental health professionals.

Cognitive Remediation

Cognitive remediation, which may use computerized games and exercises, can be helpful in improving cognitive performance, including difficulties with attention, learning, memory, and planning. As noted in Chapter 2, psychologists and other mental health professionals sometimes assess for cognitive dysfunction using a group of cognitive tests, which are also referred to as neurocognitive tests, or neuropsychological tests. Such tests might include giving the meaning of metaphors, having to follow a series of numbers or letters on a computer screen, having to spell things backward, addition and subtraction, seeing how well things are remembered after several minutes have passed, listing as many animals as possible in a one-minute period, completing a series of mazes, and similar tests. Although some of the tests can get difficult, they are often interesting to take part in if one has motivation to do so. Some of these tests also form the basis for a treatment of cognitive dysfunction: cognitive remediation. In cognitive remediation, problems with attention, memory, or other cognitive domains are improved through practice. This practice often takes place using computer programs. Some are similar to games. Cognitive remediation can take place in individual sessions, or in groups. Some of the exercises can also be done at home. Cognitive remediation is sometimes combined with other psychosocial treatments, such as supported education.

Supported Employment and Supported Education

Difficulties with employment are common for young people experiencing a first episode of psychosis. In fact, around half of people with first-episode psychosis are unemployed. However, as psychosis progresses, this figure rises to more than 75% or three-fourths of people. One way to help people with these difficulties is through a psychosocial treatment called **supported employment** (also see Chapter 13, "Going Back to School and Work"). Supported employment is one type of a more general treatment approach called *vocational rehabilitation*. Vocational rehabilitation programs provide a variety of services, including vocational counseling and guidance, assessment of work skills and interests, training in particular job skills, support services (like transportation or interpreters), and assistance with job placement. These programs help individuals with psychosis find and keep jobs. Supported employment programs help people with serious mental illnesses to work either part time or full time, while keeping their preferences at the forefront. Such programs try to place young people in the type of work that best fits them in terms of interests, skills, and comfort level. Just as supportive housing (described below) aims to move young people toward a recovery path that includes independent living, supported employment aims to move young people toward successful competitive employment (meaning a paid job) that provides them with an appropriate income.

Another approach, which is modeled closely after supported employment, is **supported education**. This psychosocial treatment supports young people with first-episode psychosis in late adolescence or early adulthood to complete their education and achieve their educational goals. Most people who develop psychosis do so at an age that interrupts their education. Furthermore, in most societies the completion of high school (if not college) is extremely important for future employment at a person's desired level. So, education is an area of psychosocial functioning that often needs attention and support. Supported education provides that.

Social Skills Training

Social skills are the daily skills that allow us to successfully interact with one another and have rewarding relationships. Developing psychotic symptoms during late adolescence or early adulthood often disrupts the process of social development and interferes with key social milestones. Young people with psychosis may have difficulties with social skills such as lacking assertiveness and finding it difficult to start a conversation.

Social skills training is a psychosocial treatment that helps individuals to improve or regain their prior level of social skills, or to resume development of social skills interrupted by psychosis. Social skills training focuses on teaching people how to approach and navigate personal and professional social situations through a combination of coaching, practicing within the clinic, getting feedback from mental health professionals or peers in the group, and then trying it out in the real world. An important part of social skills training is repetition of the targeted skill. This treatment does not necessarily focus only on symptoms. Like other psychosocial treatments, this form of treatment helps young people with psychosis move toward recovery that is broader than just reducing symptoms.

Social skills training is useful in teaching young people with psychosis to communicate successfully, interact, and become more assertive. This treatment can take place in many settings, including inpatient treatment groups, outpatient programs, and individual therapy sessions. It may be given as a single group session, as an ongoing weekly treatment, or as a part of other psychosocial treatments like CBT or group therapy.

Substance Use Treatment Programs

It is quite common for people experiencing a first episode of psychosis or another serious mental illness to have difficulties with substance use (see Chapter 11, "Staying Healthy"). Substance use usually makes symptoms worse and recovery more difficult. Young people with psychosis who are dealing with substance use have a **co-occurring disorder** (sometimes called comorbidity or dual diagnosis), which means that two disorders are present at the same time—in this case a psychotic disorder and a substance use disorder. Having both can make it harder to stick with treatment. Those with both a psychotic disorder and a substance use disorder may also have more social challenges and have increased rates of relapse. As a result, the treatment of substance use, in addition to the treatment of psychosis, is critical.

As discussed in more detail in Chapter 11, mental health professionals may recommend specific programs that target substance use. Just two examples of such programs are 12-step programs and integrated dual-diagnosis treatment programs. Alcoholics Anonymous (AA) was the first type of **12-step program**. These types of programs now exist to help people with other challenges, including the use of illegal drugs. In 12-step programs, individuals follow an ordered list of increasingly challenging tasks that take them along the road toward recovery. In these programs, someone who has completed the 12 steps often guides a newcomer just beginning the steps through the program.

An **integrated dual-diagnosis treatment program** is a treatment program that focuses on individuals who not only have a diagnosed mental illness but also have a substance use disorder. They are sometimes in an inpatient or residential setting (meaning that the young person lives there for several weeks or months). These programs treat both difficulties together at once. There are also outpatient dual-diagnosis programs in some communities. They combine, or integrate, the treatment of psychosis with the treatment of substance use in the same program. This type of treatment reduces the possibility of conflicting messages or differing treatment goals from different treatment providers.

Day Treatment Programs and Partial Hospitalization Programs

Day treatment programs and **partial hospitalization programs** are outpatient treatment facilities that provide daytime (but not overnight) treatment to individuals diagnosed with psychosis and other mental illnesses. They often serve as a "step-down" program after an inpatient hospitalization. They also may provide a more intensive treatment with an increased frequency compared to usual outpatient clinic appointments in order to prevent a hospitalization. These programs usually provide several different types of psychosocial treatments. Day treatment programs differ in the types of daily activities provided, but many of them offer a number of the psychosocial treatments discussed in this chapter. Both day treatment and partial hospitalization provide a fairly intensive form of treatment without requiring overnight hospital stays.

Assertive Community Treatment

Assertive community treatment (ACT) is a method of delivering care in which a team of mental health professionals brings treatment opportunities to people in their own settings. For example, a psychiatrist, nurse, and social worker may visit the individual in his or her home rather than in a clinic. The basic premise of ACT programs is that the treatment team comes to the young person (at home), instead of the individual having to come to the treatment team (in a clinic). They are typically designed for individuals who have difficulty managing in the community without more intensive help. Eligibility criteria may include repeated hospitalizations or safety concerns. ACT teams help people with psychosis function at their best within their own community rather than in the hospital. These teams tend to have staff members who work with fewer individuals than in other treatment settings. ACT is helpful in improving symptoms, reducing hospitalizations, and improving housing stability. There is typically no limit on the amount of time that a young person can receive ACT services, though ACT teams do help individuals transition to other services in the community when they are able to do so. Unfortunately, ACT programs are not available in all communities.

Supportive Housing

For some individuals with early psychosis, living alone or with family members is not feasible. This may be because the symptoms of psychosis interfere with their family relationships or because there are no family members available. In these cases, **supportive housing** options may be an alternative. Supportive housing provides people with serious mental illnesses a supportive and safe place to live. This could be a private apartment, an apartment shared with a roommate, or a group home. Staff members of supportive housing programs usually have knowledge of and experience with mental illnesses. However, such programs do not target symptoms directly. Instead, supportive housing focuses on assisting people with serious mental illnesses to become more independent in their living arrangements. Providing young people with this structure and support may help to decrease stress and move them toward a recovery path that includes independent living.

Putting It All Together

In addition to symptoms, young people may face difficulties in work, school, relationships, or recreation/leisure activities that often stem from the experience of psychosis. Psychosocial treatments aim to help young people overcome these difficulties and resume psychosocial development that may have been interrupted because of the time that symptoms usually appear, in late adolescence and early adulthood. Psychosocial treatments include CBT, group therapy, family interventions, cognitive remediation, supported employment and supported education, social skills training, substance use treatment programs, day treatment programs and partial hospitalization programs, ACT, and supportive housing. Mental health professionals may recommend one of these treatments or combine several depending on the individual's needs. Worksheet 8.1, which is also available in a printable form at www.oup.com/firstepisodepsychosis, can help you keep track of the psychosocial treatments that are part of your treatment plan.

Research shows that those who receive treatment early in psychosis respond better to treatment. Some have even argued that psychosocial treatments are more helpful during early psychosis than in later stages of illnesses like schizophrenia. This means that getting into effective treatment sooner may help to improve many challenges related to psychosis.

Worksheet 8.1 Psychosocial Treatments

You can use this worksheet to list the psychosocial treatments that are included in your treatment plan. It is also a place to keep the names and contact information for treatment providers.

1. Name of Treatment	Schedule
Name of Person You Will Be Working With	Contact Information
2. Name of Treatment	Schedule
Name of Person You Will Be Working With	Contact Information
3. Name of Treatment	Schedule
Name of Person You Will Be Working With	Contact Information
4. Name of Treatment	Schedule
Name of Person You Will Be Working With	Contact Information

Key Chapter Points

- The recovery process focuses as much on resuming school, work, relationships, and recreation/leisure activities as it does on treating symptoms.
- The purpose of psychosocial treatments is to help young people with psychosis overcome common challenges in these areas and resume a full life.
- Group therapy can help young people to feel less alone and give them a chance to talk to others who are going through similar difficulties and discover what's working for them.
- Family interventions help families to cope with stress, improve their social supports, and reduce the effects of stigma.
- Supported employment aims to move young people toward successful paid employment.
- Social skills training focuses on teaching people how to approach and navigate personal and professional social situations through a combination of learning new techniques and practicing these skills in various settings.

9
Follow-Up and Sticking with Treatment

When diagnosed with a first episode of psychosis, some may want to put it all behind them after leaving the hospital or clinic. Symptoms may have decreased or gone away, likely in part due to the treatment received. However, it is important to stick with the treatment plan to continue to feel better, continue to experience a decrease in symptoms, learn how to manage instances when symptoms may return, and eventually return to normal life. Mental health professionals sometimes call sticking with treatment "adherence" or "engagement."

Shared Decision-Making

Good mental health treatment places the young person and the family at the center of the treatment team and encourages active participation when making treatment decisions. Shared decision-making is a framework used by mental health professionals to ensure that the needs and preferences of young people and family members are explored and are used to guide decisions about treatment. In order to do this, the psychiatrist and other treatment team members will want everyone's input about goals for treatment, as well as preferences and individual values important to understand and respect. The mental health professionals will also share their recommendations, including the rationale for why these treatment options are recommended and the limits of treatment. Everyone is included in a discussion, listing the pros and cons of the different available treatment options. Compromise is negotiated when there is disagreement among those involved. This discussion usually leads to a consensus on how to move forward in a way that everyone can agree on. Shared decision-making can be used to plan treatment and identify goals in all settings, including the hospital or clinic.

> Shared decision-making is a framework used by mental health professionals to ensure that the needs and preferences of young people and family members are explored and are used to guide decisions about treatment.

The treatment plan will usually include (1) attending follow-up appointments with mental health professionals, (2) taking medicine as prescribed, and (3) practicing new skills. We discuss each of these as well as the importance of sticking with treatment in the following pages. However, depending on individual goals and values, the treatment plan may include other things such as getting support with school or work and decreasing use of drugs and alcohol.

Attending Follow-Up Appointments

Young people may have appointments with various mental health professionals every other week, or even more frequently, when just leaving the hospital. Those who have remained well for a longer period may have appointments less often. They may go every month and eventually only every three months. If available in the community, other choices may include appointments in the home or in the community with case managers or other mental health professionals (see Chapter 8, "Psychosocial Treatments for Early Psychosis").

Outpatient clinic appointments usually last 30 to 45 minutes. They may be with a psychiatrist or other mental health professional to check in on symptoms and how treatment is working. The individual may also benefit from counseling, therapy, or other types of psychosocial treatments. The number of appointments the young person has will depend on his or her specific goals and needs.

Not wanting to go to see a mental health professional for ongoing follow-up is understandable and normal for young people having their first experience with mental illness. However, these appointments are very helpful in many ways. For example, they allow an experienced mental health professional to hear from the young person about how they are progressing in their recovery journey and identify and address challenges and setbacks. They also allow the individual and the mental health professional to continue building a strong working relationship. And they provide a supportive environment in which young people and their families can talk about their concerns, stresses, and goals for recovery.

Taking Medicine as Prescribed

Taking medicine as prescribed is very important to help treat symptoms of psychosis. Research has proven that antipsychotics can help to relieve and reduce psychotic symptoms, sometimes completely or to a point that they do not affect daily activities. In addition to treating symptoms, medicines are also important in preventing another episode of psychosis. So, it is necessary to talk to a psychiatrist or other mental health professional rather than stopping medicine even when things are going well and the symptoms have gone away.

Like other medicines, antipsychotics may have unpleasant side effects, which differ depending on the antipsychotic taken. It is expected that young people would want to stop taking their medicines if experiencing significant side effects. By using shared decision-making, the young person can share these concerns with the psychiatrist or other mental health professional rather than stopping the medicine. They can then work together to try different medications or different dosages until they find the one that the young person can tolerate the best and benefit from the most.

It is important to understand that medicine is a necessary part of the treatment plan. Individuals with psychosis may not see the reason to keep taking their medicine once symptoms are reduced or relieved. Sometimes, they do not realize that they need medicine to keep them well or that they even have a mental health problem.

However, taking the medicine helps make recovery and pursuing one's life goals easier given that symptoms will be under better control. Furthermore, continuing the medicine reduces the chance of having a relapse and possibly having to go into the hospital. For more information on medicines, see Chapter 7, "Medicines Used to Treat Psychosis."

Practicing New Skills

Sometimes mental health professionals use certain forms of therapy in addition to medicines. Therapy, such as cognitive-behavioral therapy, and other psychosocial treatments like supported employment and social skills training give individuals various strategies and skills to practice in the real world so that the young person can learn what works for them and what does not. However, creating new habits requires practice and doing it consistently outside of the therapy sessions. This takes work and time, but if young people can practice these new strategies and skills in real-world settings with their mental health professionals or with other supports, then they will see the benefits.

How Long Treatment Lasts

How long one needs to stay in treatment will depend on individual needs and goals. Sometimes people diagnosed with a first episode of psychosis will need to be in treatment for a shorter period, but most will need to continue for months and often years. During these longer periods, it can sometimes be hard to see the success of treatment in daily life. Recovery is often not a linear process and takes time. Sticking with a treatment plan can lead to a better understanding of oneself and a better understanding of the illness and can help develop resiliency while building a meaningful life.

> Sticking with a treatment plan can lead to a better understanding of oneself and a better understanding of the illness and can help develop resiliency while building a meaningful life.

Difficulties Sticking with Treatment

Sometimes young people do not stick with their treatment plan or do not make this plan part of their daily life. Some reasons for this are:

- They may simply forget to take their medicine or attend appointments.
- They may not want a reminder of their illness by having to take medicines every day or by even talking about their illness in therapy.
- They may not see the results they expected from treatment.
- They may not believe that they have a mental health problem.
- They may distrust those around them because of certain symptoms, like paranoia, which may make them less willing to follow their treatment plan.
- They may not be able to afford their medicine and/or follow-up services.
- They may not want to deal with the side effects of the medicine.
- They may not want to give the time to attend appointments.
- They may have transportation problems that make it hard to get to follow-up appointments.
- They may lack support from others such as family and friends.
- They may be using substances regularly, which interferes with their ability to stick to their treatment plan.

Importance of Sticking with Treatment

Research has shown that young people who drop out of treatment are five times more likely to relapse with similar or more severe symptoms. This could lead to a stay in a hospital, and it may take longer to respond to treatment each time there is a relapse. Sticking with treatment is important because it decreases the chances of relapse and is the best way to prevent hospitalization. However, even people who follow their treatment plan sometimes have a relapse of psychotic symptoms. Such a relapse may be related to using substances such as marijuana (see Chapter 11, "Staying Healthy"). It may be due to stressful life events. For some people, it may be the natural course of the illness. Working with their mental health professionals, having open conversations about new or returning symptoms, and using shared decision-making to adjust the treatment plan as needed will help the young person to be better prepared should a relapse occur.

> Working with their mental health professionals, having open conversations about new or returning symptoms, and using shared decision-making to adjust the treatment plan as needed will help the young person to be better prepared should a relapse occur.

Hospitalization

Some people may decide to go to a hospital for treatment if they start to have symptoms again. In such cases, if they are hospitalized, it is called voluntary hospitalization. Others may need involuntary hospitalization if their symptoms cause them to be a threat to themselves or others or if their symptoms become severe. Involuntary hospitalization may be needed when the young person's safety or another's safety is at risk. Whether in the hospital, just coming out of the hospital, or in treatment in an outpatient clinic setting, the support of family and friends can do a lot to help people who have experienced a first episode of psychosis to stick with treatment.

Support from Family and Friends

Support from others is crucial. Sometimes people who are experiencing psychosis have impaired insight and may not fully understand their diagnosis. Family members can recognize the need for treatment and follow-up appointments when young people sometimes cannot. Family and friends should try to understand the young person's goals and treatment plan so that they can provide help and support. The worksheet at the end of Chapter 7 can help to keep track of medicines, and the worksheet at the end of Chapter 8 can help to keep track of psychosocial treatments. Both worksheets are also available at www.oup.com/firstepisodepsychosis in printable form.

Tips for Family and Friends

There are many ways that family and friends can encourage young people to stick with treatment. A few examples are:

- Make a plan with the young person for ways to help, especially if he or she starts having difficulties with taking medicine or going to appointments.
- Listen and try to be understanding of his or her issues or concerns.
- Support the young person in taking his or her medicine as prescribed and asking if he or she took it, if need be. However, it is important not to appear too controlling.
- Use helpful reminders such as a weekly pill container.
- Attend follow-up appointments with the young person.

Usually, it is best not to try to force or trick someone into taking their medicine. This could make some symptoms, like distrust or paranoia, worse, and it is not a feasible long-term option.

Support for Family and Friends

Family and friends who are supporting someone with a first episode of psychosis need support themselves. This is a difficult time, and it helps to connect with others who understand how difficult and frightening having a loved one experience psychosis can be. Mental health professionals can help family and friends to connect with others who have dealt with these same issues. These connections can be with individuals or with organizations such as the National Alliance on Mental Illness (NAMI) and Mental Health America (MHA) in the United States. Other countries have similar organizations to provide support for families and friends. These persons or organizations can provide information as well as support.

Putting It All Together

Sticking with one's treatment plan is important to continue to feel better, have fewer symptoms, and eventually get back on track with all aspects of life. Although treatment plans will differ based on individual values and goals, they usually will include attending follow-up appointments with mental health professionals, taking medicine as prescribed, and practicing new skills. While the time in treatment will differ for different individuals, most people with psychosis will need to continue treatment for a long period of time.

There are many reasons young people may not want to stick with treatment, such as not wanting reminders of the illness, possible side effects from the medicine, and time and costs of treatment. Even though sticking with treatment will be difficult at times, it decreases the chances of relapse and hospitalization and can help develop resiliency while building a meaningful life for oneself. Support both from and for family and friends is important in helping young people move toward recovery (see Chapter 14, "Reducing Stress, Coping, and Communicating Effectively: Tips for Family Members and Young People with Psychosis"). The next chapter discusses how to recognize the early warning signs of a relapse.

Key Chapter Points

- Sticking with treatment is important to continue to feel better, continue to experience a decrease in symptoms, and learn how to manage instances when symptoms may return.
- Good mental health treatment places the young person and the family at the center of the treatment team and encourages active participation when making treatment decisions.
- Shared decision-making can be used to plan treatment and identify goals in all settings, including the hospital or clinic. It can also be used to adjust the treatment plan as needed.
- Therapy and other psychosocial treatments teach individuals various strategies and skills to practice in the real world so that the young person can learn what works for them and what does not.
- Taking medicine as prescribed is important to help treat psychotic symptoms, avoid hospitalization, and make recovery and pursuing one's life goals easier given that symptoms will be under better control.
- One way that family and friends can support the young person in moving toward recovery is to understand the treatment plan so that they can help the individual stick with treatment.

PART III

HELPING YOU LOOK AHEAD TO THE NEXT STEPS

10

Knowing Your Early Warning Signs and Preventing a Relapse

In this chapter, we discuss **early warning signs**. These symptoms, though mild, may occur before the first episode of psychosis and also before later episodes. That is, some mild symptoms may occur during the prodromal phase of the illness, before psychotic symptoms first develop. These same symptoms often serve as warning signs before another episode of illness, or a relapse of psychosis, occurs. So, it is important to be familiar with early warning signs and what to do if they begin to develop.

The Importance of Detecting Early Warning Signs

Many people who have had a first episode of psychosis may go on to have one or more relapses of their illness. A relapse happens when symptoms appear again. Some relapses may happen with little or no warning over a short period of time, such as a few days. However, most relapses develop slowly over longer periods, like a few weeks. A relapse may or may not require hospitalization, but it definitely calls for immediate attention and evaluation and there will likely be changes to the treatment plan. After receiving treatment for a relapse, either in an outpatient or inpatient setting, some people feel better quickly. Others take weeks, or even months, to function as well as they had before .

One way of avoiding a relapse is to become aware of one's own specific early warning signs, which are changes in thoughts, feelings, and behaviors that start happening a few days or weeks before another episode. Early warning signs are signals that symptoms are beginning again and that another episode of psychosis may be coming. By carefully watching for these signs, young people, their families, and their mental health professionals can work together to help lessen the severity of any episode that may occur. **Relapse prevention** is best achieved by sticking with treatment, watching for early warning signs, and intervening promptly.

Relapse prevention is best achieved by sticking with treatment, watching for early warning signs, and intervening promptly.

While there are common early warning signs, they will show up slightly differently in each person. Early warning signs in one person may be clear and easy to detect, while in another person they may be trickier to figure out. The first step in determining one's own specific early warning signs is to think back to the changes that occurred in the prodromal period of the illness, or the time just before the *first* episode of psychosis.

Common Early Warning Signs

Even though each person experiences their own specific symptoms, there are some common early warning signs experienced by many people with psychosis. For some people, some of the common early warning signs we will describe (like social withdrawal, lack of motivation, and decreased expression of emotion) continue after a psychotic episode has resolved. As such, they may be long-lasting and not necessarily a warning sign for another psychotic episode. Common early warning signs include the following:

- *Mood Changes—Sadness, Tension, or Irritability:* Sadness, also called **dysphoria**, may be an early warning sign for some people who have had an episode of psychosis. They may express this sadness as feeling "down," sad, discouraged, hopeless, distressed, or uninterested in their usual activities. Tension may look like anxiety, nervousness, worry, or restlessness (such as an inability to sit still, or pacing back and forth). Some people may also come across as irritable, angry, or hostile (feeling touchy, impatient, or on edge).
- *Sleep Disturbance:* People with a sleep disturbance may have insomnia, hypersomnia, or even day/night reversal. **Insomnia** is a difficulty in falling asleep or staying asleep. For example, insomnia may mean taking more than 30 minutes to fall asleep or waking up in the middle of the night and not being able to go back to sleep. It can also be waking up more than 30 minutes earlier than one wanted in the morning. The opposite of this is **hypersomnia**, when the person sleeps more than usual. Unlike insomnia and hypersomnia, people with **day/night reversal** get about the same amount of sleep as usual but tend to stay awake at night and sleep during the day.

- *Ideas of Reference:* Ideas of reference occur when people think that others are talking about them or referring to them when they really are not. For example, a person may think that someone on the radio or the television is speaking about or trying to send coded messages to him or her. Unlike in a delusion (see Chapter 2, "What Are the Symptoms of Psychosis?"), he or she may partly recognize that these beliefs could be mistaken.

- *Suspiciousness:* People who are suspicious feel that others cannot be trusted. They may have an unexplained feeling that those around them are trying to cause problems in their life. For example, they may think that other people are plotting against them or cheating, harassing, or even trying to harm them in some way. However, unlike paranoia, they may partly recognize that their beliefs may be wrong. Even still, people with suspiciousness may begin to isolate themselves from others because they do not feel that they can trust people. An example of suspiciousness is thinking that strangers at a shopping mall are laughing at and talking about you or that someone is out to get you. It is important to remember that this is considered an early warning sign only if it is different from how the person normally behaves or thinks. Experiencing suspiciousness may be an early warning sign that more serious paranoia is about to develop.

- *Unusual Ideas:* For people to have unusual ideas as an early warning sign, the ideas must be a change from the way they normally think. People may be confused over what is real. Unlike a full delusion, people may realize that their ideas are either untrue or are an exaggeration of what is really going on. An **overvalued idea** is when too much emphasis is placed on an idea. Overvalued ideas can involve religious or philosophical thoughts, wondering about the ability to read others' minds, believing too much in superstitions, or other ideas that one is overly concerned with.

- *Trouble Thinking or Concentrating:* People experiencing this sign have problems with their thought process, or the way their thoughts work. They may become less able to organize their thoughts and speech. That is, because they are having trouble with their thinking, they may have trouble with speaking and making themselves clear. It might also be hard to concentrate, to focus their attention, or to communicate clearly with others. At times, they may have difficulty understanding what others are saying to them. They also may experience thought blocking, or an interruption in the flow of thoughts. In other words, it might be hard to put thoughts into words. As a result, they may be very slow to respond to questions or may not respond at all.

- *Perceptual Abnormalities:* A **perceptual abnormality** is when the experience of one of the five senses (hearing, seeing, feeling, tasting, or smelling) changes enough that the person wonders if their mind might be playing tricks on them. Examples include mistaking a noise for voices whispering, hearing one's name called in a noisy room, briefly seeing someone else's face when looking in a mirror, seeing something out of the corner of one's eye incorrectly, or thinking that a spot on the wall at first glance look like an object of some sort.

- *Brief, Intermittent Hallucinations:* A hallucination is a more serious form of perceptual abnormality, occurring when one senses something that does not actually exist. Examples of **brief, intermittent hallucinations** include hearing one's name called out loud that no one else hears or seeing something for a few seconds that no one else sees. Unlike a full hallucination that occurs with psychosis, a brief, intermittent hallucination happens only occasionally and lasts only a few seconds. Like perceptual abnormalities, brief, intermittent hallucinations may be an early warning sign that hallucinations are about to develop again.

- *Deterioration in Role Functioning:* A **deterioration in role functioning** is said to occur when people become less able to carry out daily activities and responsibilities. These activities can include work, school, family responsibilities, household chores, personal hygiene, recreation, and socializing. For example, there could be a drop in grades or less social interaction. Or other people might begin to notice poor hygiene. An employer may express concern that one no longer seems to be working as hard as he or she used to. These are all forms of deterioration in role functioning, which in some cases may be an early warning sign for another psychotic episode.

- *Social Withdrawal:* People who have **social withdrawal** are generally not interested in having social contact with others and are less likely to become involved socially. It can appear as if they are pulling back from social situations or that they have poor social skills. Even if they will still join in on social activities when others approach them, they tend to not seek out socializing opportunities themselves. This may happen because they feel less comfortable around others or because they are developing symptoms.

- *Low Drive, Energy, or Motivation:* People with this symptom have a significant decrease in the motivation or ability to begin and/or follow through with tasks. When lack of motivation is severe, it keeps people from finishing or completing many different types of tasks. As a result, they may neglect work, school, and/or family responsibilities. In addition, people may also stop taking care of their personal hygiene such as bathing, combing their hair, and changing their clothes. Like social withdrawal, lack of motivation may be a sign that precedes another psychotic episode. For some people, lack of motivation is a more long-lasting negative symptom.

- *Decreased Expression of Emotion:* It is important to keep in mind that normal expression of emotions differs from person to person. Normally, people express emotions through facial expressions, gestures, body language, and the tone and rate of speech. **Blunted affect** is said to occur when there is a change or lessening in their "usual" expression of emotion. While a decreased expression of emotion may be obvious to others, many people experiencing this sign are unaware of how they are presenting themselves.

- *Other Early Warning Signs:* There may be other significant changes in thoughts, behavior, or emotion that signal that a relapse of psychosis is about to happen. In general, these are things that seem "out of character" for the person. Examples of other early warning signs include not answering the phone, eating too little or too much, or making a sudden, drastic change in one's appearance.

Relapse Prevention: Responding to Early Warning Signs

It is quite common to experience one or more early warning signs just before an episode of psychosis. While there are common early warning signs, some may be unique to each person. It is important to keep in mind that each person with psychosis will not experience all of the early warning signs discussed earlier. People who have experienced an episode of psychosis should try to remember the two or three early warning signs that may be their unique signals that problems may be returning. One person's early warning signs may be insomnia, irritability, and being argumentative. Another person's may be perceptual abnormalities and brief, intermittent hallucinations. Yet another person's early warning signs may be suspiciousness and social withdrawal. It is helpful for mental health professionals, family, and other supports to be aware of the individual's particular early warning signs.

By carefully observing changes, people have a better chance of responding quickly enough to these early warning signs so that young people spend less time in the hospital—or even avoid hospitalization. Recognizing and reacting quickly to these signs is the main goal of monitoring them. There are a few important steps to take when responding to early warning signs, as discussed here and shown in Figure 10.1.

> By carefully observing changes, people have a better chance of responding quickly enough to these early warning signs so that young people spend less time in the hospital—or even avoid hospitalization.

- *Open Communication.* If it seems that early warning signs are developing, it is critical for the young person and his or her family or supports to meet to openly discuss these concerns. During that discussion, other explanations for the changes can be considered. The main goal of discussing these issues is to figure out if these changes might actually be early warning signs of a relapse. If so, it is important to begin extra measures to reduce the chance of a relapse.
- *Call One's Mental Health Professional.* The individual and his or her family should meet with their mental health professional. The psychiatrist or other mental health professional will want to meet to decide if it is necessary to temporarily increase the dose of medicine. He or she may need to draw blood to check medicine levels and will also want to assess for side effects. At times, the young person will need to switch to a different medicine. The mental health professional also may recommend adding or increasing a psychosocial treatment (see Chapter 8, "Psychosocial Treatments for Early Psychosis"). If it seems that a relapse is coming, it is important to not wait until the next regularly scheduled appointment. After noticing early warning signs, prescribing additional medicine within a few days is an important step for preventing a relapse.

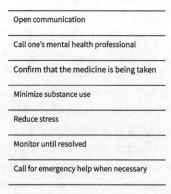

Figure 10.1 Pieces of Relapse Prevention

- *Confirm That the Medicine Is Being Taken.* Early warning signs and relapse often happen after a person has decreased his or her medicine or stopped taking medicine altogether. It is important to check the individual's medicine plan as soon as early warning signs appear. Family and friends can ask the person directly or can count his or her pills. If the person has not taken his or her medicine properly, it is time to increase reminders and encouragement for taking medicine as prescribed. At this time, it is also important to ask if the person feels that they are having any side effects that may be caused by taking the medicines, and if so, to look for a solution to side effects with the psychiatrist or other healthcare provider.

- *Minimize Substance Use.* Substance use can increase a person's risk of relapse. It is important to find out if substance use is occurring or increasing by asking the person directly and by observing the person. With increased alcohol use, he or she may smell of alcohol at times, may have poor balance or slurred speech at times, and may begin to have problems functioning. In the case of drugs, finding paraphernalia such as rolling papers, cut plastic tubes, empty vials, and small plastic bags may be a clue about drug use. Efforts should be made to minimize substance use. It is important to contact mental health professionals for their advice and help with substance use. It may be necessary to have an evaluation by a substance use counselor as well (see Chapter 11, "Staying Healthy").

- *Reduce Stress.* A person who is at risk for experiencing another episode of psychosis is often sensitive to stressful situations, such as arguments, criticism, and sudden increases in responsibility. Unfortunately, it can be difficult to evaluate stress levels because many people are not fully aware that they are under stress. It is also important to remember that stress does not cause all relapses. In addition, what is stressful for one person is not necessarily stressful for another. A person can respond to stress by reducing the source of the stress itself or by coping more effectively with the stress that exists. Reducing stress can be achieved by cutting back on responsibilities, looking for new enjoyable and relaxing activities to participate in, or dealing with a conflict or problem that is causing worry. Coping with stress can involve relaxation techniques, talking with a counselor, participating in recreational activities, or joining a support group.

> A person can respond to stress by reducing the source of the stress itself or by coping more effectively with the stress that exists. Reducing stress can be achieved by cutting back on responsibilities, looking for new enjoyable and relaxing activities to participate in, or dealing with a conflict or problem that is causing worry.

- *Monitor Until Resolved.* Once the young person and others recognize the problems and take steps to address them, it is important to monitor or watch early warning signs until there is obvious improvement. It is also important to continue meeting frequently with one's mental health professional to discuss progress. These meetings will provide important information about whether or not the young person has avoided a relapse. They also can provide information to reflect back on, if in the future there are other similar changes in behavior that are of concern. While monitoring, it is important to avoid making a person feel spied on or as if other people are "walking on eggshells" around him or her since this can be stressful. Family members should try to keep routines as normal as possible.

- *Call for Emergency Help When Necessary.* Sometimes, it may be necessary to call for emergency help if psychosis develops and the person exhibits behaviors that may be dangerous. For example, if the person threatens to harm himself or herself, or actually does something to harm self or others, it may be necessary to call for a mobile crisis team, an ambulance, or at times even police assistance. If the person is unable to care for his or her own health or safety, emergency help may be necessary. Sometimes, when psychosis develops and insight is impaired, it may be necessary for the person to go into the hospital. Most state/provincial or national governments have laws that allow doctors or the courts to hospitalize individuals against their will (involuntary hospitalization) if it is necessary in order to protect the individual and/or others. When it is necessary, hospitalization allows for more intensive short-term treatment of psychosis in a secure setting.

Putting It All Together

Even though many people who have experienced psychosis have relapses, it is possible to reduce the severity of relapses and even to prevent them. After symptoms of the first episode of psychosis go away (remission), it is important to shift the focus to not just treatment, but also relapse prevention and recovery (see Chapter 12, "Embracing Recovery"). Becoming aware of the early warning signs that are specific to a person who has had an episode of psychosis can help in monitoring for a relapse. Monitoring helps the treatment team, family, and others assist with reducing the difficulties that he or she is experiencing. By being familiar with and acting on early warning signs, a person may have less severe symptoms if a relapse does occur or may completely avoid a relapse. When responding to early warning signs, it is important to communicate openly, call one's mental health professional, confirm the person is taking their medicine as prescribed, minimize substance use, reduce stress, monitor until resolved, and call for emergency help when necessary.

Worksheet 10.1—also available in printable form at www.oup.com/ firstepisodepsychosis—will help you to record and keep track of your most likely early warning signs. It is also a place for you to keep comments and questions to discuss with your mental health professional.

Worksheet 10.1 Common Early Warning Signs

Here is a place to identify your early warning signs. Place a check next to signs that may be your early warning signs and make note of any questions or comments you may have for your mental health professional.

Common Early Warning Sign	✓
1. Sadness	
Questions or Comments:	
2. Tension	
Questions or Comments:	
3. Irritability	
Questions or Comments:	
4. Sleep Disturbance	
Questions or Comments:	
5. Ideas of Reference	
Questions or Comments:	
6. Suspiciousness	
Questions or Comments:	
7. Unusual Ideas	
Questions or Comments:	
8. Trouble Thinking or Concentrating	
Questions or Comments:	
9. Perceptual Abnormalities	
Questions or Comments:	

10. Brief, Intermittent Hallucinations	
Questions or Comments:	
11. Deterioration in Role Functioning	
Questions or Comments:	
12. Social Withdrawal	
Questions or Comments:	
13. Low Drive, Energy, or Motivation	
Questions or Comments:	
14. Decreased Expression of Emotion	
Questions or Comments:	
15. Other Early Warning Signs	
Questions or Comments:	

Key Chapter Points

- Early warning signs are mild symptoms that occur before another episode of illness, or a relapse.
- To help prevent a relapse, young people can stick with treatment, watch for early warning signs, and work with their mental health professional to intervene promptly.
- Young people can identify their unique warning signs by thinking back to the time just before the first episode to identify the two or three early warning signs that they should watch for. Family, friends, and mental health professionals can help identify the changes they observed as well.
- Open communication between the young person and his or her family, friends, and mental health professionals is important when early warning signs start to occur.
- By carefully monitoring early warning signs, young people, their families, and their mental health professionals can work together to help lessen the severity of any episode that a person may have—or prevent a relapse altogether.

11
Staying Healthy

To move toward recovery after a first episode of psychosis, young people must focus on both their mental and physical health. People with a serious mental illness are usually less healthy than those without such an illness. This may be because of certain symptoms of the illness itself (like negative symptoms) or due to not having or not going to a primary care physician. Sometimes people with a mental illness also deal with other difficulties, such as tobacco use, drug use, unhealthy eating habits, getting very little exercise, and having few relationships with others. Even though it can be difficult at times, living a healthy lifestyle is necessary for young people to feel better and move toward recovery. In this chapter, we discuss challenges sometimes faced by people with psychosis and ways to overcome them. Specifically, this chapter focuses on the importance of staying away from tobacco, alcohol, and marijuana and other drugs; having a healthy diet; getting plenty of exercise; sleeping well; and having social support from family and friends.

Staying Away from Tobacco, Alcohol, and Marijuana and Other Drugs

About one in five people in the general population in the United States (about 20%) use tobacco products. However, nearly 40% of individuals who have experienced serious psychological distress use tobacco products. Cigarettes remain the most used tobacco product in the general population compared to cigars, e-cigarettes, smokeless tobacco, and pipes. The use of e-cigarettes, vaping, and smokeless tobacco has significantly increased over the past few years and young adults are more likely to use e-cigarettes than any other adult age group.

It is estimated that about 40% of those who have a serious mental illness also have a **substance use disorder**. People receive a diagnosis of a substance use disorder when the use of a substance interferes with their ability to perform on the job, disrupts relationships, or results in legal problems, among other problems. Substances can include alcohol or other drugs like marijuana, cocaine, methamphetamine, ecstasy, heroin, ketamine, PCP, LSD, and synthetic cannabinoids. Why are people with psychosis more likely to smoke and use substances? Many mental health professionals believe that people with psychosis do this to be more social, enhance their pleasure, cope with their symptoms, or try to self-medicate.

People who smoke are at higher risk for illnesses such as emphysema, chronic bronchitis, heart disease, and lung cancer. In fact, cigarette smoking is the number one preventable cause of death in the United States and in many other parts of the world. In addition, cigarette smoking may interfere with the way the body processes some antipsychotic medicines used to treat psychosis. That is, smoking can speed up the metabolism or breakdown of some of these medicines. In other words, smoking causes some of these medicines to pass through the body more quickly. Because of this, people with psychosis who smoke may require higher doses of certain medicines to treat their symptoms. It is important to note that the chances of side effects from these medicines increase with higher doses. This is why it is important to have an open discussion about your smoking or tobacco use with your mental health professional.

As with cigarettes, there are many negative and harmful effects of using substances on the body and the brain. Drugs can affect the body and mind and coming off drugs can cause physical symptoms (like shaking, sweating, or high blood pressure) as well as psychological symptoms (like anxiety, insomnia, and irritability). Chronic alcohol use can lead to depression and liver damage and can negatively affect the metabolism of medicines, or the way they are absorbed into and work in the body. Most addictive drugs, especially marijuana, cocaine, methamphetamine, and synthetic cannabinoids, can make the symptoms of psychosis worse and interfere with its treatments. People who have experienced a first episode of psychosis are at higher risk for relapse or having another episode of psychosis if they use drugs.

Smoking cessation is the process of quitting smoking. **Nicotine replacement therapy** can be very helpful for someone trying to stop smoking. Smoking cessation programs typically offer nicotine replacement in the form of a gum, patch, lozenge, inhaler, or nasal spray (Table 11.1). These nondangerous substitutes for nicotine make it easier to reduce or quit smoking. Another treatment to help young people quit smoking is **motivational interviewing** (or **motivational enhancement therapy**), which aims—over the course of several sessions with a mental health professional—to increase one's desire or motivation to quit. Additionally, several **smoking cessation medicines**, including bupropion (Wellbutrin, Zyban) and varenicline (Chantix), are available to make quitting easier. All of these treatments

Table 11.1 Five Forms of Nicotine Replacement Therapy (NRT)

Type of NRT	Description and Availability in the United States
Gum	Nicotine is absorbed through the mucous membrane of the mouth. The gum is fast-acting and can be bought over the counter without a prescription. It is not chewed like chewing gum.
Patch	Delivers a measured dose though the skin and comes in several different types and strengths. It is available with or without a prescription.
Lozenge	Delivers nicotine through the mucous membrane in the mouth. The lozenge typically takes 20–30 minutes to dissolve and should not be chewed. It can be bought over the counter without a prescription.
Inhaler	Delivers nicotine to the mouth and is absorbed into the bloodstream. The inhaler is a thin plastic tube with a cartridge inside and most closely mimics smoking a cigarette. It is, however, not an e-cigarette. It may be the most expensive form of NRT and might only be available with a prescription.
Nasal Spray	Delivers nicotine quickly to the bloodstream as it is absorbed through the nose. The nasal spray is easy to use and relieves withdrawal symptoms quickly. However, it might only be available with a prescription.

(nicotine replacement, motivational interviewing or motivational enhancement techniques, and smoking cessation medicines) are effective at helping a person successfully quit smoking.

It is important to try to prevent substance use in people with psychosis because they are at greater risk for using alcohol and drugs. Many people with psychosis who use substances begin long before the onset or start of their illness, which may play a role in the development of psychosis in some cases. However, others begin using substances after their illness has developed to try to cope with the symptoms. Young people benefit from having someone to regularly monitor their symptoms and from frequently speaking with their psychiatrist or other mental health professionals about how they are feeling. Often, psychiatrists can adjust medicines to help the young person with psychosis feel better, and, hopefully, he or she will then not find it is necessary to turn to alcohol or drugs. Some research shows that certain types of medicines may help people with psychosis who are prone to substance use. For example, the newer, atypical antipsychotics may be more beneficial than the older, conventional antipsychotics in helping people to avoid or stop drug use. Among the atypical antipsychotic medicines, some research suggests that clozapine may be the most helpful for people with psychosis who are trying to stop using drugs.

> Young people benefit from having someone to regularly monitor their symptoms and from frequently speaking with their psychiatrist and other mental health professionals about how they are feeling. Often, psychiatrists can adjust medicines to help the young person with psychosis feel better, and, hopefully, he or she will then not find it is necessary to turn to alcohol or drugs.

Family and friends may need to help monitor symptoms. It is helpful for young people if family and friends support them through their illness and recovery. Providing a healthy, loving relationship can help them avoid drugs and alcohol. In addition, participating in healthy activities with friends can help prevent the start of substance use.

Although prevention is preferred, even those who have already begun to use substances can quit. It will be difficult, and it may take time. However, in the end, quitting will improve their mind, body, and illness. Young people should talk with their mental health professional about quitting. The mental health professional can send them to the right therapist or program to help begin and maintain this necessary change. Their mental health professional also can help them stop using substances safely, because quitting some substances suddenly, like alcohol or heroin, can be dangerous or physically painful. However, quitting can be accomplished and should be an important priority. And aside from quitting, reducing substance use is also always helpful, even if quitting is not accomplished at the time.

In some cases, a referral to a specialist, like a substance use counselor, may be necessary. A specialist may do an evaluation and make recommendations on how to best treat a substance use disorder if it is present. Such treatments may range from attending meetings (like Alcoholics Anonymous [AA] or Narcotics Anonymous [NA]), an intensive outpatient program, or even a long-term residential program, where people live in a structured recovery setting for several months or more.

Here are some steps to help someone overcome substance use:

- *Understand the change process.* Individuals often must go through stages of change to quit. These stages are becoming aware of the problem, thinking about making a change, beginning the change, and then maintaining that change long term (Figure 11.1). It is important to understand that this is a gradual process. Pushing someone to quit too quickly or being too hard on them will not help to stop the drug use. It is important for family and friends to remain supportive of the person through this process and not push them away. However, as described in Chapter 14, "Reducing Stress, Coping, and Communicating Effectively,"

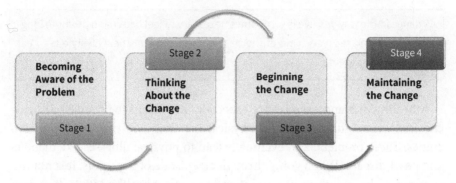

Figure 11.1 Stages of Change

family members must also maintain their own health and reduce their own stress. Some families feel that there is a point at which they can no longer tolerate some behaviors like drug use. This sometimes means that families find it necessary to take measures to get the young person into substance use treatment.

- *Keep communication open.* The young person has to feel comfortable and free to talk about the difficulties of quitting. This open communication provides much-needed support. It also allows family and friends a chance to express their concerns about the young person's well-being and future. For someone who is in the change process, having others to turn to can be extremely helpful.

- *Provide support at every possible opportunity.* Finally, young people need support in other ways when trying to quit using substances. For example, they may need someone to attend appointments or AA or NA meetings with them. Supporting the young person also can help family and friends to learn what is happening and how to best help the young person in managing his or her illness and use of drugs.

Having a Healthy Diet and Getting Plenty of Exercise

A healthy diet and frequent physical exercise should be part of everyone's life. These two things are necessary for a strong, healthy body and mind. People with an illness especially need to focus on taking care of themselves, and this is true for any sort of illness. A change in the way you live is sometimes necessary to feel better and promote long-term health and recovery. One of the best ways to start this new lifestyle is to eat healthier and to exercise.

A change in the way you live is sometimes necessary to feel better and promote long-term health and recovery. One of the best ways to start this new lifestyle is to eat healthier and to exercise.

A healthy diet and exercise are especially important for people with psychosis. Overweight/obesity and physical inactivity are two common difficulties. These problems can eventually lead to physical illnesses like diabetes and heart disease. When going through an episode of psychosis, it is not uncommon to be less physically active and to neglect healthy eating. It may be difficult to be physically active and maintain healthy eating habits because of symptoms such as low drive, energy, or motivation, and some side effects of medicine such as increased appetite. Antipsychotic medicines also can cause metabolic side effects. For example, they can sometimes cause elevations in blood glucose and cholesterol levels. Weight gain and metabolic side effects must be carefully monitored by the psychiatrist or other healthcare provider because if these occur, they can increase one's risk for future diabetes or heart disease. Some ways the psychiatrist may monitor for weight gain and metabolic side effects are discussed in Chapter 7, "Medicines Used to Treat Psychosis."

Changing the way one eats and starting an exercise plan can be overwhelming at times. Start small by setting achievable weekly goals and track progress along the way to keep motivated. Websites from the U.S. Food and Drug Administration and the USDA MyPlate program can provide further information and resources when making changes toward a healthier diet.

Here are a few suggestions for eating well and thus feeling good:

- *Eat a colorful plate.* Increase the amount and types of fruits and vegetables you eat. Fill half of your plate with colorful fruits and vegetables at every meal.
- *Make half of your grains whole grains.* Add more whole grains to your diet by setting a goal of making half of the grains you eat whole grains. Examples of whole grain products include whole wheat bread, whole wheat pasta, oatmeal, popcorn, and brown rice.
- *Hydrate the healthy way.* Drink more water and less sodas, juices, or sports drinks. Sodas, juices, and sports drinks can contain high amounts of sugar. Start cutting down on sodas by replacing one bottle that you would normally drink with one large glass of water. Seltzer or soda waters are also alternatives to soda. Just make sure that there is no added sugar if buying flavored water.

- *Do some exercise every day.* Exercise for at least 30 minutes a day at a moderate intensity, five days a week. Examples include brisk walking, mowing the lawn, or bicycling at a light effort. Many gyms have free trials for new members, so try something new until you find an exercise program that is right for you.
- *Spread out your workouts.* It can be hard to find the time to exercise for one long period. Instead, spread your workouts over the day. Aim to exercise for at least 10 minutes at a time.
- *Walk when you can.* If you are taking public transportation, get off one stop early. If you are driving, park farther away. Also, take the stairs when you can. Every extra step adds up.
- *Work out with others.* Find a friend or family member to work out with or join a group fitness class. Working out with others is a great way to stay motivated.

Sleeping Well

Another common issue for young people experiencing psychosis is difficulty with sleep. Good sleep is essential to both mental and physical health. According to the National Academy of Sleep Medicine, adults aged 18 to 60 years need seven or more hours of sleep per night, and teens aged 13 to 18 years need even more, at eight to ten hours. Even when some get this amount at night, they might have poor sleep quality. Examples include not feeling rested after waking and waking up multiple times during the night.

Good sleep habits are essential to getting the amount and quality of sleep one needs. Such habits include consistently going to bed and getting up at the same time every day, not using electronics for 30 minutes to one hour before bed, leaving cellphones and other electronics in another room at night, eating lighter meals at night, and not drinking caffeine after lunch. If sleep problems continue, seek advice from your psychiatrist or other mental health professional.

Having Good Social Support from Family and Friends

For young people to make these necessary lifestyle changes, they will need support from family and friends. Having the support of family and friends is good for one's mental health and physical health. People who have support from others enjoy longer, healthier lives. There are many benefits to having social support from loved ones. These benefits are extremely helpful to people experiencing an episode of psychosis. For example, spending time with others can help to reduce stress. Because stress can trigger symptoms, reducing stress may decrease symptoms or decrease the risk of relapse.

> Having the support of family and friends is good for one's mental health and physical health. People who have support from others enjoy longer, healthier lives.

It can be hard to keep relationships with friends or form new relationships with others when going through an episode of psychosis. This is understandable. One reason is that young people have to deal with symptoms that cause problems with socializing. They may have trouble communicating, a lower attention span, or no interest in talking with others. Their ability to trust others may also be affected. These and other problems can make it hard to get close to others.

It is important to strengthen existing relationships with family and friends. Young people experiencing psychosis should be encouraged to connect with others and should not be overly protected or restricted. People who have had an episode of psychosis still occasionally become frustrated or angry and need to complain, like everyone else. A supportive environment will allow them to express these emotions without overreacting. Everyone needs help, especially when going through difficult times.

Young people with psychosis might think it is hard to find friends who understand and accept them. Developing close, supportive friendships is possible; one should not give up. Others may be more open than one might expect. Young people can look to organizations or groups for new connections. Some possible places could be community or church groups. One can also turn to the local chapter of the National Alliance on Mental Illness (NAMI) or Mental Health America (MHA) in the United States, or to similar support organizations in other countries.

Putting It All Together

A healthy lifestyle is necessary to begin to feel better and move toward recovery. A healthy lifestyle includes not using tobacco products, alcohol, or drugs (or reducing use); having a healthy diet and exercise routine; sleeping well; and having social supports. Starting this journey might be difficult, and it might be tempting for someone to turn to substances or away from the help of others.

Mental health professionals can recommend certain therapies, such as nicotine replacement therapy, motivational interviewing or motivational enhancement therapy, or smoking cessation medicines, to help one quit smoking. Treatments for quitting substance use may range from attending regular support meetings, to an intensive outpatient program, or even a longer-term residential program. Again, discussing options with mental health professionals is important to safely quit using alcohol or drugs.

Other common challenges that affect people with psychosis are overweight/obesity, physical inactivity, and poor quality of sleep. A healthy diet, regular exercise, and sleeping well are important to fight against heart disease, diabetes, and weight gain caused by some medicines. This can be difficult because of certain experiences common with an episode of psychosis. However, support from family, friends, mental health professionals, and those who have dealt with psychosis themselves can help one succeed. Everyone needs help from others at times, and this is no different for those experiencing psychosis. Keeping up relationships with friends and family and forming new relationships is important.

Key Chapter Points

- To move toward recovery after a first episode of psychosis, young people must focus on both their mental and physical health.
- Staying away from tobacco products, alcohol, and marijuana and other drugs; having a healthy diet; getting plenty of exercise; sleeping well; and having social support from family and friends are all necessary parts of a healthy lifestyle.
- Even those who have already begun to use substances can quit, and though difficult, in the end quitting will improve their mind, body, and illness. Even if not ready to quit, reducing substance use is always helpful.
- One way to change the way one eats and to start an exercise plan is by setting achievable weekly goals and tracking progress along the way to keep motivated.
- Good sleep habits are essential to getting the amount and quality of sleep one needs. These include going to bed and getting up at the same time every day, not using electronics for 30 minutes to one hour before bed, leaving cellphones and other electronics in another room at night, eating lighter meals at night, and not drinking caffeine after lunch.
- Young people with psychosis might think it is hard to find friends who understand and accept them. Developing close, supportive friendships is possible; one should not give up.

12
Embracing Recovery

When someone recovers from a physical illness, others often think of him or her as cured. But what about in the field of mental health? At present, there is no cure for some mental illnesses that cause an episode of psychosis, such as schizophrenia. So, what does it mean for a person with a mental illness to be in recovery? One way of thinking about recovery is that instead of people recovering *from* a mental illness, they recover *despite* the mental illness. In other words, people can develop meaningful activities and relationships while learning to manage and live with their mental illness.

Recovery is different from **remission**. Remission means that the major symptoms, usually positive symptoms like hallucinations and delusions, are no longer active. The goals of remission and recovery go hand in hand. But recovery is a much broader concept, pertaining to one's life goals, rather than to just getting symptoms under control. Some people experiencing psychosis may appear to recover completely. Others may require ongoing work to improve to the greatest possible level of recovery despite having a long-term illness.

The Recovery Model of Mental Health Treatment

The **recovery model** of mental health treatment is a change in thinking about treatment and living with a serious mental illness. Before, to most people, the word *recovery* meant that an individual was symptom-free or improved to some point set by mental health professionals. In the new way of thinking, recovery begins by focusing on the person's life goals rather than about the illness alone, then moves into helping the person figure out how they want to be a part of and contribute to the community and larger society. Individuals themselves decide on their personal goals—and have a major voice in treatment planning, along with family members—instead of mental health professionals making decisions alone. Recovery involves an individual reaching his or her goals for independent living, employment, social relationships, and community participation. People with mental illnesses want to have meaningful relationships, and to give something to their communities. Increasing an individual's skills and functioning through mental health treatment is a major part of the recovery process.

The goal of the recovery model of mental health treatment is to empower individuals to achieve their fullest potential in life. The recovery philosophy embraces the belief that one can achieve life goals when given freedom, support, necessary information, education, high-quality and specialized services, and the opportunity to develop skills, have rewarding jobs, and be in meaningful relationships.

> The recovery philosophy embraces the belief that one can achieve life goals when given freedom, support, necessary information, education, high-quality and specialized services, and the opportunity to develop skills, have rewarding jobs, and be in meaningful relationships.

There is no single definition of recovery. People also have different opinions on what type of recovery plan would work best for individuals with serious mental illnesses. The recovery model of mental health treatment recognizes and honors the individual, which ultimately translates into the person having decision-making power in his or her care. Mental health professionals who embrace the recovery model agree that this is the best way to help the individual achieve whole health and a fulfilling life.

Principles of Recovery

Some basic ideas about recovery include (Figure 12.1):

- *There are many pathways to recovery.* Just as each person's symptoms and life situations are different, each person's journey in recovery will be

Many pathways to recovery

Self-directed and empowering

Personal recognition of the need for change

Holistic

Takes into account cultural dimensions

Continuum of health and wellness

Figure 12.1 Principles of Recovery

different as well. Recovery focuses on each individual and what best fits his or her life.

- *Recovery is self-directed and empowering.* Since each person is different, the individual decides what is most important to him or her. These goals are the starting point for recovery plans. For example, if getting a job is most important to that individual, then supported employment might be a critical service. Because individuals decide in conjunction with their mental health professional and their family using shared decision-making, they can have a strong voice in planning for their future.
- *Recovery requires a personal recognition of the need for change.* Others should not force individuals to change. Only the young person can decide if a change is necessary for his or her life.
- *Recovery is holistic and based on strengths.* Recovery focuses on mind, body, relationships, activities, and environment. A person must look at all parts of his or her life when deciding how best to achieve individual goals.
- *One's culture is important in recovery.* When thinking about the whole person, it is necessary to understand his or her cultural background. Understanding a person's culture can clarify an individual's beliefs or attitudes toward his or her illness and recovery. Mental health services that are recovery oriented should also be culturally sensitive.
- *Recovery involves health and wellness.* As noted before, recovery does not focus on reducing symptoms alone. Recovery involves much more, such as physical health, self-awareness, functioning in desired roles, life satisfaction, self-esteem, and wellness. The nature and quality of the health and wellness of a young person depend on how it is defined by the individual and his or her capacity and desire to achieve personal goals.
- *Recovery is not a linear process.* The recovery process may be a lifelong process with ups and downs. There may be many accomplishments, as well as some setbacks, during recovery.

> Recovery focuses on mind, body, relationships, activities, and environment. A person must look at all parts of his or her life when deciding how best to achieve individual goals.

The recovery model of mental health treatment emphasizes the individual's own desires and decisions. This does not go against mental health professionals' recommendations for treatment. Rather, the recovery model aims to strengthen the sharing of decisions between young people experiencing psychosis, their families, and mental health professionals. Research has shown that medicines and psychosocial treatments are very helpful. This is why mental health professionals often strongly encourage young people to stick with these treatments. However, in more recent years, people experiencing psychosis and their families have shown mental health professionals that they want to be more involved in their own treatment decisions. The recovery model supports this call for a greater voice in planning treatment and setting goals.

Characteristics of Being in Recovery

Recovery in mental health may be a lifelong process. It requires learning, support, courage, and patience. As with any other illness, recovery in a mental illness can have ups and downs. People in recovery maintain a positive attitude and a sense of hope for their lives. However, they realistically understand that their lives may be different from before. They are aware that it may now be necessary to deal with symptoms and setbacks. Their lives have changed, but they are ready for the challenges ahead.

People in recovery find and capitalize on their strengths and accept themselves. This is often coupled with an ability to take charge of their lives. Part of recovery for many people is to return to work or school, reconnect with others, or live independently. More people recover in psychosis than is often realized.

> People in recovery find and capitalize on their strengths and accept themselves. This is often coupled with an ability to take charge of their lives. Part of recovery for many people is to return to work or school, reconnect with others, or live independently. More people recover in psychosis than is often realized.

While the individual is ultimately in charge of his or her own recovery, having the support of others during this journey is extremely important. It is very helpful to communicate one's needs to family, friends, peers who are also in recovery, mental health professionals, and community members. This allows others to give support and work together with the individual to identify his or her strengths, analyze the existing barriers, and enhance chances of achieving goals.

Peer Specialists, Peer Support, and Reducing Stigma

Others have learned to live with their illness and have full, happy lives through recovery. People who are successfully living with psychosis, including peer specialists (sometimes also called peer counselors or peer navigators), can help support others with psychosis because they have had their own journey in recovery. The importance of incorporating peer specialists as employees in mental health treatment teams has become increasingly recognized in recent years.

Coordinated specialty care programs (as described in Chapter 5, "Finding the Best Care") are also recognizing the crucial role that peer specialists can have in supporting young people experiencing psychosis for the first time. Many are now offering **peer support** (from peer specialists) as a part of their services. In addition to finding peers in an increasing number of outpatient mental health programs, there are also peer organizations and groups throughout the United States and other countries where young people can find support.

One element of peer support and the vital role of peer specialists pertains to fighting or reducing **stigma**. Stigma is a form of discrimination that stems from lack of understanding about mental illnesses. Peer specialists, because of their own lived experience, and in their role as a staff member working within the treatment team, can help reduce stigma and negative stereotypes in the clinical setting and in the larger community as well.

Putting It All Together

Recovery means successfully living with a mental illness by not being confined by it; embracing hope, empowerment, and self-determination; and focusing on one's personal life goals and roles in society. It differs from remission because it focuses on more than just symptom control. Instead, recovery focuses on personal goals decided by individuals themselves. Some basic principles of recovery are that there are many pathways to recovery, it is self-directed and empowering, it requires a personal recognition of the need for change, it is holistic and strengths-based, it considers cultural backgrounds, and it involves whole health and wellness.

Individuals may have setbacks at times. Recovery is a process of learning and patience. One has to think of the whole person—mind and body—to be in recovery. It is an attitude and a way of life. By embracing this empowering philosophy, many people live in recovery and have deeply meaningful lives.

Key Chapter Points

- Recovery is a broad concept, pertaining to one's life goals, rather than to just getting symptoms under control.
- The goal of the recovery model of mental health treatment is to empower individuals to achieve their full potential in life.
- Individuals themselves decide on their personal goals for treatment and recovery instead of mental health professionals deciding for them.
- Recovery requires learning, support, courage, and patience.
- People who are successfully living with psychosis, including peer specialists (or peer counselors or peer navigators), can help support others with similar experiences because they have had their own journey in recovery.

13
Going Back to School and Work

Finishing high school, going off to college, and getting a first job are major milestones in a young person's life. These milestones are visible signs of adult independence and set the foundation for future employment, income, and achievements. They also offer important opportunities to form lasting social connections for an individual's personal and career development. Because of the typical age when psychosis develops, interruptions in school and work are common. Such issues can often be seen even in the prodromal phase before the symptoms of psychosis begin. Because of this, rates of school dropout and unemployment are higher in those experiencing a first episode of psychosis. However, experiencing an episode of psychosis does not change young people's goals. They are the same as for any other peer. They want to go to school, get a job, have friends, have a romantic relationship, and live on their own. These are the same goals that any of us would have at that age.

The Importance of School and Work

The importance of staying in school and having a job is commonly recognized in programs designed to serve young people experiencing psychosis. In coordinated specialty care programs, described in more detail in Chapter 5, "Finding the Best Care," there is usually a staff member solely dedicated to support clients to achieve goals in these two areas, school and work. In fact, one of the key outcomes used to measure the success of coordinated specialty care programs is the number of clients who gain competitive employment (which means a paid job) and/or enroll in school. This is because we know that the longer someone is out of work or school, the harder it is for them to go back.

Going to work and earning a paycheck—or going to school and passing classes while learning important information for a future career—will help an individual to feel productive and confident, increase social connections, and enhance self-esteem. Coordinated specialty care programs try to get young people back to work and school as soon as possible. Though some people, including some mental health professionals, may think that this would be too stressful for someone who has just experienced a first episode of psychosis, one model of supported employment which coordinated specialty care programs often use (called Individual Placement and Support) has shown the benefits of more rapid return to school or work.

> Going to work and earning a paycheck—or going to school and passing classes while learning important information for a future career—will help an individual to feel productive and confident, increase social connections, and enhance self-esteem. Coordinated specialty care programs try to get young people back to work and school as soon as possible.

Supports for Going Back to School and Work

The **Individual Placement and Support (IPS)** model was developed in the 1990s at Dartmouth University as a means of supporting employment goals for individuals diagnosed with serious mental illnesses. As such, it is a type of personalized support often referred to as supported employment (or supported education when the focus is on going back to school). Since its development, the IPS model has been found to be more effective and to produce better outcomes than other employment programs for individuals with serious mental illnesses. Some of its principles include zero exclusion (meaning that anyone interested in getting a job is eligible for services), rapid engagement and employment, a focus on competitive (meaning paid rather than volunteer) employment, being integrated with the rest of the treatment team, continuing support after getting a job, and valuing clients' own preferences.

In the IPS model, anyone who wants to work is eligible for services even if symptoms are still present or if the individual is not taking medicine. IPS employment specialists support the individual through the entire process of writing a strong resume, searching for a job, and going on interviews, and even after the person has started working, as the person may still need support navigating and coping on the job. The goal of IPS is to have an individual actively searching for a job and beginning the interview process as soon as possible. Individuals apply to jobs open to any other candidate, including individuals who do not have mental illnesses, and jobs applied to are based on one's own preferences and interests. Employment specialists counsel individuals on disability benefits and the options for work, if the person is receiving such benefits. In addition, IPS employment specialists actively build relationships with potential employers in the community. Expanding on the

IPS model for employment, coordinated specialty care programs also add educational support for those wishing to return to high school or go to college. For educational support, enrollment in mainstream education becomes the focus of the support services.

If supported employment or supported education services are not available in one's community, there are other opportunities for support. If employment is the goal, one place to start would be to search for a resume building workshop or class, and then see what other sessions or supports are available from those programs. Career interest inventories are useful to identify and explore possible career goals. Since many young people have never been employed and are looking for their first job, support in identifying goals and interests in work can be valuable. A job fair is also a great opportunity to see what's available and meet potential local employers.

> Since many young people have never been employed and are looking for their first job, support in identifying goals and interests in work can be valuable.

For educational goals, colleges offer regular campus tours that are usually student-led and will allow an opportunity to see what the campus culture and environment are like. GED programs are available in most areas for those who did not finish high school and wish to pursue that option. Also, vocational programs are an option for those interested in learning a trade. As with employment, tools such as career interest inventories can be helpful when identifying areas of study and degrees one would be interested in pursuing.

A young person's mental health professional should also be involved in decisions around returning to work or school, in conjunction with the family. Even if they are not specialists in supported education and supported employment, mental health professionals can offer important help to ensure a young person achieves his or her goals for education and employment. For example, they can help the young person with coping strategies for situations that may come up at school or on the job. A psychiatrist can prescribe medicines for certain symptoms and experiences that may be getting in the way of success.

Mental health professionals may also offer cognitive tests or psychological testing that can assist in identifying weaknesses as well as strengths and can be helpful when developing goals for work and school. For employment goals, mental health professionals can offer ongoing support throughout the job-seeking process, which can be challenging due to the need to maintain motivation while coping with possible rejection (i.e., not getting a specific interview or job). Mental health professionals can also help to support family members who may have concerns about educational and employment goals and can help the family come to a shared decision and form a plan to move forward. Family members and friends are the most important supports a young person has during this transition back to school or work, and it's important to strengthen those supports.

> Mental health professionals can help to support family members who may have concerns about educational and employment goals and can help the family come to a shared decision and form a plan to move forward. Family members and friends are the most important supports a young person has during this transition back to school or work, and it's important to strengthen those supports.

Points to Consider

If a young person decides that they want to pursue educational or employment goals, there are a few options to consider. Should the young person pursue both at the same time, or just one? Some young people move between wanting to focus on school or work, and others want to pursue both at the same time. Should the young person plan to start working or going to school part time or full time? It may be easier to start part time until the young person feels comfortable to move up to full-time work or school. If one decides not to pursue school or work even part time, there are volunteer opportunities through community organizations that could provide experience in an area of career interest while deciding on future plans for school or work. Is the young person receiving disability benefits or planning to apply for benefits? If so, it is important to understand when and how employment will affect benefits. Talking with a mental health professional can help to better understand the rules in an individual's home state or province. Sometimes one can work a certain number of hours or earn a certain income before government benefits are reduced.

Certain services are available to those with a disability in an educational setting and certain rights are guaranteed by law in a work setting. For example, an **Individualized Education Plan** (IEP) is a plan developed in elementary, middle, and high schools for a student with a disability to ensure they are receiving the additional supports necessary for academic success. College campuses typically have an Office of Student Services that can also provide extra supports for students with disabilities.

Telling Others About One's Mental Illness

Whether or not to tell others about one's mental illness is something that every young person who experiences psychosis will likely think about and make decisions around, especially when preparing to go back to a previous job, return to school, or start in a completely new job or school. It is a personal choice. There can be different levels of disclosure that the young person may choose. A young person may choose to tell others that they have a mental illness but not the specific diagnosis, or they may choose to disclose that they have a disability but not say that it is a mental illness. Young people who have had a recent first episode of psychosis may not be ready to disclose their recent experiences in a school or work setting or may not identify with certain labels.

The individual also decides what his or her mental health professional will disclose. In most countries, for a mental health professional to be able to discuss anything about an individual's illness or treatment, or even whether or not they are working with that individual at all, a release form must be signed by the individual if 18 or older, or by their parent or guardian if still a minor. The individual decides what can be released unless they are at risk of harming themselves or others.

Putting It All Together

Finishing school and working at a meaningful job are goals that most young people have, which set the stage for future career and personal achievements. Unfortunately, difficulties at school and work are common for someone experiencing psychosis and there may have even been difficulties beginning before the symptoms of psychosis. Family and friends may worry that returning to school or work may be too stressful for the young person. If the young person's goals center around education and employment, there are options and supports for returning to the classroom or workplace that the individual and his or her family should discuss with their mental health professional. Models such as IPS have shown that rapid return to employment produces better outcomes, and coordinated specialty care teams have incorporated supported employment and supported education services as one of their core offerings. Going to work, or doing well in school, gives one a sense of purpose and achievement. These are important steps in recovery that can be achieved with the right supports from family, friends, and mental health professionals.

Key Chapter Points

- Finishing high school, going off to college, and getting a first job are visible signs of adult independence and set the foundation for future employment, income, and achievements.
- Though some may think that going back to school or work could be too stressful for a young person who has recently experienced a first episode of psychosis, one model of supported employment, IPS, has shown the benefits of more rapid employment.
- Expanding on the IPS model of supported employment, coordinated specialty care services add educational support, as many young people wish to get back into school or pursue both work and school goals.
- If one decides not to pursue work or school immediately, there are volunteer opportunities through community organizations that could provide experience in an area of career interest while deciding on future plans for school or work.
- Whether or not to tell others that one has a mental illness is a personal choice and one that every young person who experiences psychosis will make decisions around, especially when preparing to go back to a previous job, return to school, or start in a completely new job or educational activity.

14

Reducing Stress, Coping, and Communicating Effectively

Tips for Family Members and Young People with Psychosis

As discussed in previous chapters, psychosis often first begins in late adolescence or young adulthood. Because of this, many people who experience a first episode of psychosis live with and rely on their families for support. In addition to providing a place to live and other basic resources, families are key in the recovery process because they love the person with the illness, care for them, and want to help.

Family members may need to provide emotional support, arrange for treatment, and find new ways to cope with the symptoms of psychosis (see Chapter 2, "What Are the Symptoms of Psychosis?") or other problems that result from the illness. With effective antipsychotic medicines (see Chapter 7, "Medicines Used to Treat Psychosis") and psychosocial treatments (see Chapter 8, "Psychosocial Treatments for Early Psychosis") available, many people with psychosis receive treatment in the community and with their families. Families are a very important part of the team and play a major role in helping their loved ones manage their psychosis. As a result, it is vital to create a supportive family environment by reducing stress, promoting healthy coping, and communicating effectively.

This chapter focuses on three essential domains of a supportive family environment: (1) reducing stress, (2) enhancing coping, and (3) ensuring effective communication. First, we begin by defining stress and the ways that the early stages of psychosis can lead to stress. We discuss three ways to reduce stress in the family as well as three related ways the family can help the young person with psychosis to reduce stress. Second, we define coping and discuss the importance of coping with a stressful event, like an episode of psychosis in a loved one. We offer three ways of coping effectively for family members as well as three ways that young people can practice effective coping. Third, we address the value of good communication and how the symptoms of psychosis can sometimes interfere with productive communication patterns. We then provide points of advice for effective communication within the family.

What Is Stress?

The word **stress** describes a feeling of strain, pressure, or tension. Some stress is a normal part of life, and every person and family experiences stress. **Stressors** are events that cause stress. In general, there are two types of stressors: life events and ongoing stressors. **Life events** include things such as becoming ill, experiencing the death of a loved one, going through a divorce, getting married, having a baby, getting a new job, or moving. Some life events are more stressful than others. It is important to remember that whether a life event is positive or negative, it can still bring about stress. In addition to life events, **ongoing stressors** are a part of everyone's life. Some of these include frequent or repeated arguments or conflicts, financial problems, constant criticism, being unemployed, or a chronic illness in a loved one.

Stress can have a wide range of effects on people. These may include physical changes (such as muscle tension or headaches). Stress can also lead to changes in thinking (such as concentration problems), mood (such as irritability, anxiety, or depression), and behavior (such as restlessness, angry outbursts, or substance use). Learning to manage stress in a healthy way is essential to everyone's physical and mental health.

Stress and the Early Stages of Psychosis

When someone experiences an episode of psychosis, they feel stressed. It is also normal for family members to feel very stressed when a person in their family experiences an episode of psychosis. Family members may find the process of the initial evaluation, the diagnosis, and treatment choices to be stressful, overwhelming, and confusing. However, just as one person can pass stress to another, reducing one family member's stress helps to reduce stress for the whole family. So, working together to develop better ways of handling stress strengthens relationships and improves the quality of life for everyone in the family.

For some people who have experienced psychosis, stress may trigger a relapse (see Chapter 10, "Early Warning Signs and Preventing a Relapse") and even hospitalization. It is essential then that the family, as well as the young person's mental health professionals, help him or her with ways to reduce stress. Improving the young person's ability to manage stress helps to decrease his or her risk of relapse.

Ways to Reduce Stress in the Family

There are many ways to reduce stress within the family as a whole; three examples follow (Figure 14.1).

- *Learn about psychosis.* Families that educate themselves about psychosis are better able to solve problems and support their loved one. They are better able to reduce stress, cope well, and communicate effectively. This, in turn, can help the young person's illness. Chapter 8 discusses how family interventions, including family psychoeducation and family therapy, can be a vital part of the treatment plan. Learning about psychosis requires that the family be comfortable asking questions of their mental health professionals. Families also can learn about dealing with psychosis and reducing stress by talking to other families who have a loved one with a psychotic disorder.

> Families that educate themselves about psychosis are better able to solve problems and support their loved one. They are better able to reduce stress, cope well, and communicate effectively.

- *Set reasonable expectations.* The key is to have balance by avoiding extremes. Family members need to set reasonable expectations for themselves. For example, it is not possible to constantly remain by the young person's side to provide support and monitoring. A balance is needed between monitoring and giving him or her enough space to recover and live a self-directed life. Family members need to stay engaged in their own lives by making use of support from friends, enjoying hobbies, participating in exercise, and caring for their own physical and mental health.
- *Make time for enjoyable family activities.* It is important for families to continue to do activities together that they normally enjoy and prioritize time together as a family. They may do outdoor activities like a picnic, go to the park or lake, attend sporting events, watch a movie, or simply share a family meal together. Family activities may be especially helpful when dealing with serious stress, such as psychosis in a loved one.

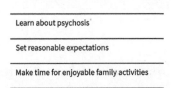

Learn about psychosis

Set reasonable expectations

Make time for enjoyable family activities

Figure 14.1 Ways for Families and Young People to Reduce Stress

Ways for People with Psychosis to Reduce Stress

There are many ways that people with psychosis can reduce stress and many things that families can do to help. Examples of activities that may help reduce stress, based on the same three general themes just listed for the family, are described next.

- *Ask questions about your illness.* Just as families need to learn about psychosis, so does the person experiencing psychosis himself or herself. As discussed in Chapter 8, psychoeducation is an essential part of the treatment plan. Like families, young people should feel comfortable asking their mental health professionals questions about psychosis and treatments.
- *Find the right balance.* Just as it is helpful for families to set reasonable expectations, the same is true for the person experiencing psychosis. Again, the key is to have balance and to avoid extremes. For example, for someone who has recently experienced an episode of psychosis, working or going to school full time may be too demanding at first. However, not working at all may lead to boredom, unhappiness, lack of fulfillment, or financial problems. So, working part time could be fulfilling, give a sense of purpose, and provide some financial relief. The importance of returning to school or work, whether part time or full time, was detailed in the previous chapter. Reasonable expectations also need to be set for other goals, such as returning to school, finding a partner, and having a child.
- *Enjoy hobbies and recreation.* Just as enjoyable family activities can help reduce stress within the family, hobbies, recreation, and other fulfilling activities are important for young people with psychosis. For some people, work or school is enjoyable. Others may enjoy being involved in their faith community, volunteer activities, music, exercise or sports, reading, or the arts (artwork, music, theater, dance). These, as well as many other activities that bring pleasure, are valuable for reducing one's level of stress.

What Is Coping?

The word **coping** refers to facing and dealing with stress, problems, or difficulties in a successful and healthy way. It is important to keep in mind that one cannot avoid all stressors. Some are a natural part of trying to fulfill personal goals and of life. Making a plan to enhance one's coping strategies, or ways of dealing with stress effectively, is very important. Within the family, family members should figure out what type of coping strategies each person uses and enhance them to the extent possible. Similar attention to coping strategies is helpful for the young person.

> Making a plan to enhance one's coping strategies, or ways of dealing with stress effectively, is very important. Within the family, family members should figure out what type of coping strategies each person uses and enhance them to the extent possible.

How Family Members Can Cope Effectively

Included next are three ways, among many other possibilities, to help families cope with and manage the stress of psychosis in a loved one (Figure 14.2).

- *Talk and think positively.* The more negatively a person views something, the more stressful it may feel. Many people have self-defeating thoughts when faced with a difficult situation: "This is horrible," "I hate this," or "I won't succeed." Better thoughts to replace these are "I'm going to give it my best try," "While it's not my first choice, I can deal with it," or "It's a challenge, but I can handle it." While changing one's point of view may not get rid of the stressor, it can reduce its impact. Family members can talk and think positively to prevent feeling overwhelmed or defeated by their loved one's psychosis. Consistent with the advice to think positively, the recovery model of mental health treatment itself focuses on empowerment, optimism, hope, and determination (see Chapter 12, "Embracing Recovery").
- *Take care of yourself.* It can be tiring and emotionally draining to care for someone with a mental illness like psychosis. Given the stress of dealing with psychosis in a loved one, it is easy for family members to forget to take time for themselves or even to neglect their own needs. To be most

Talk and think positively

Take care of yourself

Embrace your spirituality or other supports

Figure 14.2 How Family Members Can Cope Effectively

helpful for their loved one, family members must be healthy—both physically and mentally. It is important to take care of oneself through regular exercise, a healthy diet, leisure activities, and good social support. Family members benefit from reducing their own stress and seeking care for themselves when it is needed.

- *Embrace your spirituality or other supports.* Faith communities and religious beliefs help many people cope with stress when faced with difficult situations. For some people, prayer and other religious activities may greatly reduce stress. Other community groups also can provide social support, which can help one to feel less isolated and stressed. Also, support can often be found by including other extended family members in one's support network.

How Young People with Psychosis Can Cope Effectively

There are many ways to go about effectively coping with having an illness that causes psychosis; three things that may help cope with the stress of psychosis are described next (Figure 14.3).

- *Practice relaxation.* Several techniques can lessen the effects of stress on mental and physical health. Some examples include breathing exercises, progressive muscle relaxation, mindfulness practices, meditation, and yoga. Books, apps, classes, online videos, or sessions with trained professionals are all ways to learn these techniques. When first learning a technique, it will be necessary to concentrate on doing the steps, but as the steps become familiar, it will be easier to relax.
- *Maintain good health habits.* Eating a healthy diet and getting enough sleep can provide the strength to deal with stress. Regular physical exercise can decrease stress, improve sleep, and increase well-being. Almost any physical activity has a positive effect on reducing stress, improving sleep patterns, and lifting mood. It is also important to avoid unhealthy

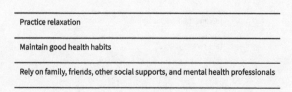

Practice relaxation

Maintain good health habits

Rely on family, friends, other social supports, and mental health professionals

Figure 14.3 How Young People with Psychosis Can Cope Effectively

habits, like smoking cigarettes, drinking alcohol excessively, and using drugs. Maintaining healthy habits is not only good for long-term health, but it also supports coping with current problems. For more on the importance of good health habits, see Chapter 11, "Staying Healthy."

- *Rely on family, friends, other social supports, and mental health professionals.* Social supports are good for one's physical and mental health. The support that family members, friends, and others in your community can provide is vital for coping with a serious illness. Additionally, mental health professionals are very knowledgeable about various treatment options and helping people to find their own best ways of reducing stress and coping with the illness.

The Importance of Communication

When people are feeling stressed, no matter the stressor, effective communication often breaks down. Coping with psychosis can be a major stressor for everyone involved. It can be especially challenging when the family provides most of the care and support for the person experiencing psychosis. Good communication can lower the amount of stress and conflict in the family. Lower family stress and conflict can help to decrease the possibility of future negative outcomes of the illness. It also can reduce the risk of relapse and improve symptoms. Effective communication is helpful in all relationships, including relationships among family members, especially during times of stress.

Symptoms of Psychosis Can Sometimes Interfere with Communication

Some symptoms of psychosis can make communication between family members and the person who is experiencing psychosis difficult at times. Being able to recognize when symptoms are making communication difficult helps family members to respond appropriately. Some reasons why symptoms may make communication difficult are described next.

- *Positive symptoms can make it difficult for the young person to know what is real and what is not.* Positive symptoms like hallucinations and delusions are distracting and can be frightening. Hallucinations can be too difficult to ignore while speaking and may interfere with communication.

The voices may even tell the person experiencing psychosis not to talk or to say things that are inappropriate. Family members should realize that hallucinations are very real to the person experiencing them. The voices are not imagined or made up. Delusions can also interfere with communication. For example, some delusions may cause people to think that anything they say becomes evidence that others are using against them. They may think that a police agency is recording their conversations. Regardless of what the delusion is about, family members should not try to disprove or talk the person out of the delusion. They also should not go along with the delusion given that it does not represent reality and going along with the delusional belief would be dishonest. Paranoia also can interfere with trusting others or feeling safe about expressing thoughts and feelings. It may be helpful to try to empathize with the young person by taking time to understand what it would feel like to have these troubling experiences.

- *Negative symptoms can make it difficult for family members to know how their relative is feeling.* For example, blunted affect (such as when the face does not show emotion), anhedonia (reduced ability to experience pleasure), and apathy (not caring as deeply) are often misinterpreted as being lazy or giving up. Not knowing how the person feels can make a conversation very difficult. Family members should realize that these negative symptoms are not under the person's control but result from the illness causing the symptoms of psychosis. Sometimes negative symptoms also make it difficult for people experiencing psychosis to recognize other people's feelings, causing people to miss nonverbal cues, such as facial expression and tone of voice.
- *Disorganization can cause confusion when trying to communicate successfully.* Disorganized thoughts do not make logical sense. The person sounds confused or comes across as confusing. People experiencing this symptom can go so far off topic that they may take a very long time to make a point. At other times, family members may have communication problems because of their loved one's unclear, meaningless, or unchanging responses. Being slow or unable to respond to questions also makes communication challenging. It is helpful for family members to be very clear and straightforward when talking with their loved one with disorganized thoughts. Patience is very important.
- *Cognitive (thinking) problems can cause misunderstandings because of difficulties in concentrating, making decisions, or remembering things.* Someone experiencing psychosis may need more time to think about what someone is saying to figure out how to respond. Often, people give up on them for taking too long or wrongly think the delay is a sign of disinterest.

Advice for Effective Communication within the Family

Improving communication can improve the overall quality of life for the entire family. Effective communication helps to reduce relationship problems, resulting in fewer conflicts and unresolved disagreements.

Improving communication can improve the overall quality of life for the entire family. Effective communication helps to reduce relationship problems, resulting in fewer conflicts and unresolved disagreements. This will reduce the level of stress for the family and result in fewer emotional problems for everyone. Included next are eight ways to effectively communicate in the family that are sensitive to the challenges posed by symptoms of psychosis (Figure 14.4).

- *Be brief and stick to the point.* Keep communications simple and direct, avoiding difficult language. Getting to the point will lessen misunderstandings. Often, people tell all the details of an entire event to help make the story more interesting and to make sure that they do not leave anything out. When talking to someone with psychosis, however, it is better to make sure to communicate just what one needs to share. For example, instead of saying, "I was going to the bank, because I needed some money to buy your prescription, and I ran into your cousin. She has a new haircut and was dressed very professionally. Anyway, I didn't find out what sort of work she's doing now, but she did tell me to say 'hello' to

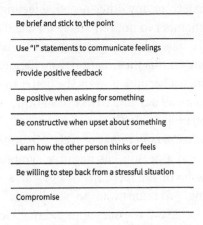

| Be brief and stick to the point |
| Use "I" statements to communicate feelings |
| Provide positive feedback |
| Be positive when asking for something |
| Be constructive when upset about something |
| Learn how the other person thinks or feels |
| Be willing to step back from a stressful situation |
| Compromise |

Figure 14.4 Advice for Effective Communication Within the Family

you," it may be better to say just, "I ran into your cousin today, and she asked me to say 'hello' to you."

- *Use "I" statements to communicate feelings.* Verbally expressing both positive and negative feelings lessens the need to guess about what the other person is feeling. This leads to less confusion and tension even when expressing something that is upsetting. One way to do this is by using "I" statements. Instead of referring to someone else (e.g., "Your uncle thinks you need to wash your hair more often") or asking questions (e.g., "Don't you think you should wash your hair tonight?") it may be better to use "I" statements such as, "I am worried that you aren't washing your hair as often as you used to."

- *Provide positive feedback.* Often, people with a psychotic disorder feel as if they cannot do anything well anymore. It helps to hear that others are proud of them for something or pleased by something they have done. They will come to understand what their own personal strengths are, instead of focusing only on their limitations. Giving loved ones compliments that are brief and specific encourages them to realize their strengths.

- *Be positive when asking for something.* People who have experienced psychosis may be sensitive to criticism and hostility. Nagging and demanding usually leads to resentment, hurt feelings, and a tendency to be uncooperative. It helps to use brief, specific "I" statements in a calm, pleasant voice. For example, instead of saying, "Get to that bedroom of yours already and clean it," or "You're such a slob" it would be better to say, "I would feel better about our home if you would clean your bedroom."

- *Be constructive when upset about something.* Everyone gets upset with others at one point or another. When expressing sadness, frustration, anger, worry, anxiety, or any other negative feelings, it helps to be brief and specific. Remember to not rely solely on facial expressions and tone of voice. Verbally state what is upsetting and then offer suggestions for correcting it or preventing the situation from happening again. Instead of saying, "You're such a hermit," it would be better to say, "I'm worried that you sit in your room all day, and I'd like to sit down and think about some activities that you might enjoy."

- *Learn how the other person thinks or feels.* Misunderstandings and frustration can occur if a person has negative symptoms and others must guess about how he or she feels. Instead of guessing, ask. For example, rather than saying, "You don't want to be with me," it would be better to say, "You hardly came out of your room today. I'd feel better if you could tell me how you feel about spending time with me." Family members should verify what the person is saying by restating what they heard and asking if they understood correctly. For example, if the young person says, "Those people might hurt me," the family member then might say, "So, it sounds like you feel unsafe because of those people you have been thinking a lot about. Is that right? How can I help you to feel safer?"

- *Be willing to step back from a stressful situation.* Avoid unnecessarily staying in a stressful or emotionally charged conversation. Taking a break often allows both people to have the chance to calm down so that they can better communicate and solve problems later. It would be helpful to say something like, "Our conversation is stressing me out right now. I'd like to take a break and take a walk so that I can calm down and be better able to talk about this situation later."
- *Compromise.* In a compromise, each person usually gets something that he or she wants but also must give up something. The ultimate goal is to reach a decision that is acceptable to both people. When a compromise occurs, it is a "win–win" situation.

Putting It All Together

Families are a very important source of support for young people who are trying to manage an episode of psychosis. People who have experienced psychosis and their families can work on creating a supportive family environment by reducing stress, coping, and communicating effectively. It is understandable and expected that young people and families would feel stress during an episode of psychosis. However, it is important to reduce stress, which may trigger a relapse or even rehospitalization. Both families and young people can reduce stress by learning about psychosis, setting reasonable expectations, and making time for enjoyable family activities.

Because it is impossible to get rid of all stress in one's life, it is important to develop ways to cope with stressors that may occur. Young people with psychosis and their families can use several strategies for coping effectively such as staying positive, taking care of themselves, and seeking support. Stress in a family can sometimes start to break down communication between family members. Certain symptoms can also make communication difficult at times. Good communication can reduce stress, lower conflict, and reduce the risk of negative outcomes. Specific strategies can help improve communication within the family, such as being brief and concise, using "I" statements when communicating feelings, providing positive feedback, being positive when asking for something, being constructive when upset, learning how the other person thinks or feels, being willing to step back when faced with stressful situations, and compromising.

Mental health professionals may recommend family therapy or family psychoeducation, two valuable psychosocial treatments briefly described in Chapter 8. Research has shown that these family interventions reduce relapse and hospitalization, improve outcomes, and enhance adjustment. Additionally, family members will benefit from seeking information on psychosis, including support that can be gained from organizations such as the National Alliance on Mental Illness (NAMI), Mental Health America (MHA), and similar organizations in other countries.

Key Chapter Points

- Families are key in the recovery process because they love the person with the illness, care for them, and want to help.
- It is vital to create a supportive family environment by reducing stress, coping, and communicating effectively.
- It is impossible to get rid of all stressors because some are just a natural part of life or trying to reach personal goals.
- Learning to manage stress is important to everyone's mental and physical health.
- Working together to develop better ways of handling stress strengthens relationships and improves the quality of life for everyone in the family.
- Effective communication helps to improve relationships, resulting in fewer conflicts and unresolved disagreements.

15

Understanding Mental Health First Aid for Psychosis

Throughout this guide, we have tried to explain all parts of a first episode of psychosis in a detailed way. But what happens if you know someone who may be experiencing an episode of psychosis and you have to act fast or help them get into treatment? This last chapter includes advice on how to provide mental health first aid to those who may be experiencing an episode of psychosis. These guidelines were developed by and reprinted here with permission from Mental Health First Aid Australia. They created these guidelines based on the expert opinions of people with lived experience of psychosis (individuals with psychosis and their family members) and mental health professionals (clinicians, researchers, and educators) from Australia, Canada, Germany, Ireland, the Netherlands, New Zealand, Sweden, Switzerland, the United Kingdom, and the United States. For more information on their Mental Health First Aid program, please visit www.mhfa.com.au. The remainder of this chapter is organized around questions addressed to help people who may need to provide first aid to someone experiencing psychosis.

Purpose of These Guidelines

These guidelines are designed to help members of the public to provide first aid to someone who may be experiencing psychosis. The role of the first aider is to assist the person until appropriate professional help is received or the crisis resolves.

How to Use These Guidelines

These guidelines are a general set of recommendations. Each individual is unique, and it is important to tailor your support to that person's needs. So, these recommendations may not be appropriate for every person.

How Do I Know If Someone May Be Developing Psychosis?

It is important to learn about the early warning signs of psychosis (see Chapter 10, "Early Warning Signs and Preventing a Relapse") and the symptoms of psychosis (see Chapter 2, "What Are the Symptoms of Psychosis?"). A single symptom does not necessarily indicate that someone is experiencing psychosis. However, psychosis is more likely if there is a group of symptoms, or changes that are very out of character for the person. The symptoms of psychosis may appear suddenly or develop or change gradually over time and can vary from person to person. They can be triggered by a range of factors, such as extreme stress or trauma, or there may not appear to be a trigger at all. A person may experience psychosis as a single episode or as part of an ongoing illness and can experience multiple episodes of psychosis with periods of complete or partial wellness in between. It is also important to consider the spiritual and cultural context of the person's behaviors, as what is interpreted as a symptom of psychosis in one culture may be considered normal in another culture. Some things to avoid doing are given in Figure 15.1.

How Should I Approach Someone Who May Be Experiencing Psychosis?

A person developing psychosis may not reach out for help. If you are concerned about someone, approach them in a caring and nonjudgmental manner. You should approach them for a one-on-one conversation, rather than a group discussion. Do this in an environment that is likely to be safe, comforting, and free of distractions. Allow adequate time to have a conversation with the person.

Do not ignore or dismiss warning signs, even if they appear gradually or are unclear. For example, a change in motivation or interest in life could be a symptom of psychosis returning.

Do not assume that a person exhibiting symptoms of psychosis is 'just going through a phase', is a 'teenager being a teenager', or that they are experiencing the normal ups and downs of life, or misusing substances.

Do not assume that any symptoms of psychosis will go away on their own.

Figure 15.1 Things to Avoid If You Think a Person May Be Experiencing Psychosis

A person developing psychosis may not reach out for help. If you are concerned about someone, approach them in a caring and nonjudgmental manner.

Try to be calm, regardless of the person's emotional state. Do not approach the person in a confrontational manner. If you are concerned about how the person will react to your approach, consider having a support person nearby. Tailor your approach and interaction to the way the person is behaving. For example, if they are suspicious and avoiding eye contact, you should be sensitive to this and give the person the space they need. If the person approaches you because they want to talk about what they are experiencing but you do not have time to give them your full attention, you should explain this to them and offer to meet when you can give them more of your attention.

How Should I Talk to the Person About What They Are Experiencing?

The person may be aware of what is happening to them, may have no insight at all, or may not accept that they are unwell. Start by trying to find some common ground for discussion, gradually building up toward more specific questions about what the person is experiencing. Do not use the term "psychosis," but rather discuss any concerning changes in thoughts, feelings, or behavior that you have noticed in the person.

Ask the person if they want to talk about how they are feeling or explain what they are experiencing. Allow them to talk about their experiences, feelings, and beliefs in order to gain an understanding of their perspective. As far as possible, let the person set the pace and style of the interaction. Be aware that the person may be vague when describing their symptoms and may emphasize physical symptoms over symptoms of mental illness. Acknowledge the courage it may have taken for them to talk to you.

If the person has noticed changes in their behavior, ask them how long they have been experiencing these and if they are distressed by them. Tell the person that you understand they may be frightened by what they are experiencing. Do not tell the person that you understand completely what they are experiencing and do not speculate to the person about a diagnosis. If there are other people present, do not speak about the person as though they are not there.

When talking to the person about what they are experiencing, follow the tips for communicating in Table 15.1.

Table 15.1 Tips for Communicating with a Person Who May Be Experiencing Psychosis

Language	Use everyday rather than simplified language.
	Use language that normalizes the person's experience, such as the word "stress."
	Use the same terminology that the person uses to describe their experiences.
	Do not use stigmatizing terms.
Listening Nonjudgmentally	Convey empathy when communicating with the person and listen to them nonjudgmentally.
	Acknowledge what the person is saying and how they are feeling: "That sounds really upsetting" or "It sounds like you don't know what to do."
	Listen carefully to the person, reflect what you hear, and ask clarifying questions to show that you are listening.
	Recap what the person has said to check that you have understood correctly.
Body Language	Do not touch the person without their permission.
	Minimize body language that shows distress or nervous behavior such as shaking one's legs, fidgeting, or nail biting.
	If the person is sitting down, do not stand over them or hover near them.

How Can I Be Supportive and Understanding?

Ask the person if, and how, they would like you to support them. Reassure them that you are there to help and want to keep them safe. Also, ask them if there are any current stressors that may be contributing to their symptoms, and whether they would like practical support such as assisting them with medical appointments. However, do not try to immediately provide the person with solutions. You should make it clear to the person what you are willing and able to do to support them.

Social support can be helpful for the person. However, the person may lack social support because they isolate themselves or their behavior leads others to withdraw from them. If appropriate to the relationship and situation, ask the person if it is okay to check in with them from time to time, and if it is, continue to reach out to the person to let them know you are thinking about them and that you care. If you do have ongoing contact with the person, watch for signs that indicate they may be experiencing a worsening of their symptoms. However, in these ongoing interactions do not focus only on the person's mental health problems. Also, it is important to avoid being negative or pessimistic when talking to the person about their future.

Social support can be helpful for the person. However, the person may lack social support because they isolate themselves or their behavior leads others to withdraw from them. If appropriate to the relationship and situation, ask the person if it is okay to check in with them from time to time, and if it is, continue to reach out to the person to let them know you are thinking about them and that you care.

How Can I Treat the Person with Dignity and Respect?

It is important to always treat the person with respect. You should support the person in making their own decisions about their mental health and not attempt to take over or make decisions for the person without their involvement. Accept that the person may not follow suggestions you make.

Avoid using patronizing or trivializing statements when interacting with the person, such as "Cheer up," "I'm sure it will pass," and "It could be worse." Do not tell the person to get their act together. Be tolerant of changes in the person's behavior, unless their behavior becomes dangerous or inappropriate. Do not express anger or frustration you may feel toward the person. If the person is upset by something you have said or done, you should apologize and acknowledge their feelings. Unless the person is a danger to self or others, you should respect their privacy and right to confidentiality.

How Should I Respond to Delusions and Hallucinations?

It is important to know that delusions or hallucinations are very real to the person. Ask the person if they want to talk about what they are seeing or hearing. If the person wants to talk about their hallucinations or delusions, you should listen, show empathy, and develop an understanding of what they are experiencing. When talking to the person, you should use their own terminology when referring to hallucinations or delusions, such as "the voices" or "your worries about your safety."

It is important to try to empathize with how the person feels about their beliefs and experiences, without stating any judgments about the content of those beliefs and experiences. You should acknowledge to the person that what they are experiencing is real to them, without confirming or denying

Do not pretend to agree with the person's hallucinations or delusions.
Do not try to reason with the person about their hallucinations or delusions.
Do not dismiss, minimize, or argue with the person about their hallucinations or delusions.
Do not act alarmed or embarrassed by the person's hallucinations or delusions.
Do not laugh at or make fun of the person's hallucinations or delusions.
Do not ridicule the person, even if what they are saying does not make sense to you.

Figure 15.2 What *Not* to Do When Responding to Someone with Hallucinations or Delusions

their hallucinations or delusions. You could do this by stating, "I accept that you hear voices or see things in that way, but it's not like that for me."

If the person is hearing voices, they may respond to the voice they are hearing by talking or whispering to themselves. Remember that the person is experiencing symptoms that are beyond their control and you should not blame them or take their actions personally. Some things not to do when someone is responding to hallucinations or delusions are given in Figure 15.2.

You should ask the person if there is anything they have found that reduces their hallucinations or delusions, and if there is, encourage them to use these strategies if they are healthy and adaptive. Ask them if they are afraid or confused. If it is appropriate to the relationship, let the person know you love and support them, as this can help them to feel safe. If you observe other people making jokes about or criticizing the person, you should tell them to stop.

What If the Person Is Experiencing Paranoia?

People's experience of hallucinations or delusions may cause them to not trust people, even those close to them. If the person is experiencing paranoia, you should:

- Tell the person that you do not see any threats, but that you will stay with them if it helps them feel safe.
- Encourage and support them to move away from whatever is causing their fear, if it is safe to do so.
- Tell the person what you are going to do before doing it—for example, that you are going to get out your phone.

- Give the person simple directions, if needed, such as "Sit down, and let's talk about it."
- Stay with the person, but at a distance that is comfortable for both of you.

Do not encourage or inflame the person's paranoia, such as by whispering to or about them. Likewise, do not use body language that could exacerbate paranoia. For example, do not approach the person with your hands in your pockets or behind your back, or stand over or too close to them.

What If the Person's Communication Is Affected?

A person experiencing psychosis may not be able to communicate in the way they normally would and their level of comprehension and capacity to reason may be affected. For example, they may respond with unrelated answers or drift from one topic to another. Hearing voices may also make it difficult for them to communicate because they are distracted. They may miss nonverbal cues such as facial expression and tone of voice. If appropriate and feasible, you should check with others who know the person for advice on the best way to communicate with them.

You should try to communicate clearly and simply, repeating things where necessary. Avoid using complex language such as metaphors or sarcasm. It is important to allow the person enough time to respond to questions or statements, as they may have difficulty processing information.

If the person's speech has become disorganized, focus on the person's feelings rather than what they are trying to say. If they are showing a limited range of feelings, be aware that it does not mean that this is all they are feeling. Likewise, do not assume that the person cannot understand what you are saying, even if their response is limited. If the person is having trouble communicating, you should know that your presence alone can be reassuring for the person.

How Do I Respond to Challenges During the Discussion?

Even if the person realizes they are unwell, their confusion and fear about what is happening to them may lead them to deny that there is anything wrong. If the person denies anything is wrong or does not wish to talk about what they are experiencing, do not argue with them, insist they are unwell, or try to force them to talk. It is important to know that several conversations may be necessary before the person is open to talking to you.

Focus on listening rather than trying to change the person's mind. Do not threaten consequences in an attempt to change the person's behavior. Ask the person if there is anything specific you can do to help them and let them know that you will be available to talk in the future. If the conversation with the person becomes stressful or emotionally charged, you should take a break to allow yourself and the person to calm down.

> If the person denies anything is wrong or does not wish to talk about what they are experiencing, do not argue with them, insist they are unwell, or try to force them to talk. It is important to know that several conversations may be necessary before the person is open to talking to you. Focus on listening rather than trying to change the person's mind.

You should be aware that the person may react with emotions that don't seem to fit the context of the conversation, such as laughing. If you find the person's behavior annoying or irritating, understand that the situation may be distressing to both of you.

Professional Help

How Should I Encourage the Person to Seek Professional Help?

Convey a message of hope by telling the person that help is available and things can get better. To encourage the person to seek professional help, tell them that:

- What they are experiencing could improve with appropriate professional help.
- Seeking professional help as soon as possible is important because early treatment is more effective and can prevent symptoms from getting worse.
- Seeking professional help does not necessarily mean they will be hospitalized, as early treatment can take place in the community.
- Health professionals will have the person's well-being and best interests in mind.
- Health professionals must maintain confidentiality except in limited circumstances, such as if the person is at risk of harming self or others, or if directed to disclose information to a court.

- It is okay to seek help, and this is a sign of strength rather than weakness or failure.

Try to find out what type of professional help the person believes will assist them and provide them with a range of options for seeking professional help. However, if the person is having trouble making decisions, limit the number of options you offer them.

Ask the person whether they have a doctor they trust, and if they do, you should encourage them to make an appointment with their doctor. Another reason to encourage them to see their doctor for a checkup is because symptoms of psychosis may stem from physical illnesses. If you find out the person is not taking their prescribed medication, encourage them to talk to their doctor about it.

Do not threaten, confront, or put pressure on the person when encouraging them to seek professional help. Be aware of the influence that the person's family may have. For example, the family may encourage or discourage the person from obtaining the care that they need. However, if the person is an adolescent and you have a duty to care for them, ensure that they get an appointment to see a health professional and offer to go with them. If the person asks for advice or suggestions regarding treatment, tell them that they should talk to a health professional about these.

How Should I Support the Person to Get Professional Help?

Reassure the person that you will support them while they seek and receive professional help. If the person has an appointment, ask them if they would like you, or another relative or friend, to accompany them to their appointment. Continue encouraging the person to seek professional help, even if challenges arise in the process of obtaining care. If the person is having difficulty getting advice or help, encourage them to contact a mental health advocacy or support agency.

What If the Person Does Not Want Professional Help?

If the person does not want to seek professional help, remain patient, as people experiencing psychosis often need time to recognize or accept that they are unwell. Explore the reasons why the person does not want to seek professional help. These may include not realizing they are unwell, worries about stigma, not knowing where to get help, or because they believe that others are trying to harm them.

Calmly express your concern to the person about their choice to not seek help and the potential implications. Ask them what they think the pros and cons of seeking professional help would be. Stress the potential benefits of getting help, such as relief from anxiety or frightening symptoms.

Focus on trying to find something that the person agrees is a problem and then suggest that they seek help for that. For example, if they say that they feel anxious around other people, you should encourage them to seek help for anxiety.

If the person does not recognize that they are unwell, they might actively resist your attempts to encourage them to seek help. Be prepared to have several conversations with them before they are willing to seek professional help.

The person has the right to refuse treatment, unless they meet the criteria for involuntary treatment. You should be aware of state/provincial and national laws relating to this. However, you should never threaten someone with involuntary treatment or hospitalization. Let the person know about other options for help in their community. It is important to try to maintain a good relationship with the person, as they may want your help in the future.

If the person does not want to seek professional help, you may wish to discuss your concerns about the person with a health professional. If you do so, clearly describe your observations (meaning exactly what the person has been doing and saying, where, and when) so that they have all the necessary information. However, while you are entitled to express your concerns about the person to their health professional and ask for their assistance, the health professional must maintain confidentiality about the person unless the person has granted consent or is a minor (and you are their legal guardian).

What About Self-Help Strategies and Other Supports?

Ask the person if they have felt this way before, and if so, what they have done in the past that has been helpful. Encourage the person to try self-help strategies, such as relaxation methods, physical activity, and good sleep habits. You should encourage the person to look after their physical health by maintaining a healthy lifestyle and getting regular medical checkups.

Try to determine whether the person has a supportive social network and, if they do, encourage them to use these supports. Ask the person if they want to talk to family or friends about what they are experiencing. Encourage them to talk to someone they trust.

What If the Person Has Recently Given Birth?

Postnatal psychosis is a condition in which symptoms of psychosis begin suddenly within the first few weeks after giving birth. Postnatal psychosis can escalate rapidly and delays in treatment can lead to increased risk for the mother and her baby. If you think a mother may be experiencing postnatal psychosis, or is having delusions about her baby, call a mental health crisis team immediately. Try to involve the mother's partner or family in minimizing any risk to the mother or baby. Ensure that someone is with the mother and baby at all times until professional help is received.

What If the Person Has Been Using Alcohol or Drugs?

Discourage the person from misusing alcohol or drugs, and tell them that these may worsen symptoms of psychosis. If the person has been using alcohol or drugs, do not blame or lecture them about this. If you think the person has been misusing alcohol or drugs, you can follow the "Mental Health First Aid Guidelines for Helping Someone with Alcohol Use Problems" and the "Mental Health First Aid Guidelines for Helping Someone with Drug Use Problems." These can be downloaded from www.mhfa.com.au.

What If the Person Is in a Severe Psychotic State?

A person is in a severe psychotic state if they have overwhelming delusions or hallucinations, very disorganized thinking, or bizarre and disruptive behaviors. They may appear very distressed, their behaviors may be disturbing to others, or they may behave in a way that endangers themselves or others. They may or may not behave aggressively. Aggressive behavior may range from verbal abuse to physical abuse and can cause physical or emotional harm to others.

Safety Considerations When the Person Is in a Severe Psychotic State

If you think the person may be in a severe psychotic state, approach them with caution. Be aware that the person might act on hallucinations or delusions. Your primary goal should be to keep the person, yourself, and others safe. Stay at a safe distance from the person while being able to maintain interaction and ensure you have clear access to an exit. It is important to assess for risk of harm to the person or others, and take any threats or warnings seriously, particularly if the person believes they are being persecuted. If you are frightened, seek outside help immediately, as you should never put yourself at risk.

If safe to do so, try to limit access to means that the person could use to harm self or others by removing any weapons, or objects that could be used as weapons, from their immediate environment. If the person has a weapon, you should not approach them and should call emergency services immediately.

De-escalation When the Person Is in a Severe Psychotic State

Do more listening than talking. Allow the person to express their feelings and empathize with them. Speak to the person in short, simple sentences, and use direct questions. Speak calmly and do not raise your voice or shout at the person. Try to minimize the level of emotion you show; remain calm and do not show fear or anxiety. Try not to take anything they say personally.

Do not do anything to further agitate the person. Avoid nervous behavior such as shuffling your feet, fidgeting, making abrupt movements, or talking fast. If it is necessary to move close to or make physical contact with the person, you should first ask them for permission. For example, you could ask, "Do you mind if I sit next to you?" or "I can see your arm is hurt. Is it okay if I use the first aid kit to bandage it?"

Ask the person whether they would like you to decrease distractions and stimulation by turning off the TV or reducing room lights. If there is more than one person present, try to create a space around the person so that they don't feel crowded. Encourage only one person to speak at a time and do not argue with any other people present about the best course of action. Do not try to restrict or restrain the person's movement.

Try to gather information about whether the person feels safe by stating, "You seem worried. Is there anything I can do to help?" or "Do you feel safe? Is there something you are afraid of?". Let the person know you are there to help. Ask them what you can do and attempt to find out what would help them feel safe and in control. If the person has a **psychiatric advance directive** or relapse prevention plan, you should follow this. Try to find out if the person has anyone they trust, such as close friends or family, and if so, try to enlist their help. If you are not able to de-escalate the situation, call for professional assistance such as a mental health crisis service or emergency services.

Seeking Help When the Person Is in a Severe Psychotic State

Try to make sure the person is evaluated by a health professional immediately. Explain to the person why you believe that a medical or mental health assessment is necessary. Provide the person with options regarding seeking professional help, as this may give them a sense of control. For example, "Do you want to go to the hospital with me or would you prefer John to take you?" If the person has been receiving professional help for psychosis, encourage them to contact their health professional. If you need to contact a mental health service, do not label the person's problem as "psychosis," but rather outline any symptoms and immediate concerns.

If your concerns about the person are dismissed by the services you contact, persevere in trying to seek support for the person and call another service. If you are alone with the person and cannot stay, call someone to stay with the person until professional help arrives.

If you suspect the person may be a risk to self or others, contact emergency services immediately. However, do not use calling emergency services as a threat. If you need to call emergency services, explain that the person is in urgent need of medical help. Be aware that the person won't necessarily be admitted to the hospital. If you think the person is at risk of suicide or harming themselves, tell emergency services this. Explain that you are concerned the person may be experiencing psychosis. Describe specific, concise observations about the person's behavior and symptoms. If the person has previously been diagnosed with a psychotic illness, you should explain this. Let the emergency services know if the person is armed or if there are accessible weapons nearby.

> If you suspect the person may be a risk to self or others, contact emergency services immediately.

If emergency services respond, try to meet them on arrival so you can explain the situation before they approach the person. If the police respond, be prepared that the person may be restrained or face charges. As other people arrive, explain to the person who they are, that they are there to help, and how they are going to help.

If the Person Is in a Severe Psychotic State and Needs to Go to the Hospital

If you think the person needs to go to the hospital, but do not feel it is safe for you to take them, call emergency services. If the person goes to the hospital, and it is appropriate to the relationship, you should try to speak directly to the doctor or emergency staff to provide information relevant to the person's situation. If the person needs to be admitted to the hospital, support them by focusing the conversation on how a hospital stay might bring relief by reducing their symptoms.

What If the Person Appears to Be Behaving Aggressively?

People with psychosis are not usually aggressive and are at a much higher risk of harming themselves than others. Do not make assumptions about whether the person will be aggressive or not, but be aware of potential risks to others. Certain symptoms of psychosis (for example, visual or auditory hallucinations, or paranoia) can cause people to become aggressive and the person's aggression may be driven by fear.

Do not threaten the person, as this may increase fear or prompt further aggressive behavior. Do not respond in a hostile, disciplinary, argumentative, or challenging manner. Avoid asking the person too many questions, as this can spark defensiveness and further anger them. If the person becomes aggressive, this may be made worse by certain steps you take, such as involving the police.

If the police are called, tell them that the person may be experiencing psychosis and that you need their help to obtain medical treatment and to control the person's aggressive behavior. Let the police know whether or not the person has a weapon. If you are alone with the person, call someone else to accompany you until professional help arrives. If the person's aggression escalates, remove yourself from the situation.

What If I Think the Person Is at Risk of Suicide?

If you think the person is at risk of suicide, you can follow the "Mental Health First Aid Guidelines for Suicidal Thoughts and Behaviors." These can be downloaded from www.mhfa.com.au.

If you do not think the person is at immediate risk of harm, but are still concerned about their welfare, ask the person if there is someone close to them who may be able to support them to stay safe. If the person is an adolescent and they want to contact a parent or other trusted adult, offer to stay with them while they do so.

How Can I Look After Myself?

You may feel a range of emotions (shock, confusion, or guilt) when you realize someone close to you is experiencing symptoms of psychosis. These are common reactions. It is also common to experience negative feelings (fear, sadness, anger, or frustration) as a result of supporting a person who is experiencing psychosis. You should look after your own mental health and well-being. Do not put pressure on yourself to find solutions to all of the person's problems. If you are finding your role stressful, seek support for yourself through support groups and organizations, a health professional, or a supportive friend, while maintaining confidentiality. Try self-help strategies to reduce any stress you experience, such as relaxation methods, regular exercise, enough sleep, and a healthy diet.

> Do not put pressure on yourself to find solutions to all of the person's problems. If you are finding your role stressful, seek support for yourself through support groups and organizations, a health professional, or a supportive friend, while maintaining confidentiality.

Key Chapter Points

- Each individual is different, and it is important to tailor your support to that person's needs.
- You should recognize that the individual may be frightened by their thoughts or hallucinations. Ask the person about what will help them to feel safe and in control.
- The person may refuse to seek help even if they realize that they are unwell.
- You should be aware that the person might act on paranoia, a delusion, or hallucinations. Remember that your primary task is to de-escalate the situation, so you should not do anything to further upset the person.
- If the person is at risk of harming themselves or others, you should make sure that mental health professionals evaluate the person immediately.
- If you are frightened, seek outside help immediately. You should never put yourself at risk.
- When contacting the appropriate mental health service, you should not assume the person is experiencing a specific psychiatric illness but should instead explain the symptoms, behaviors, and immediate concerns.
- The role of the first aider is to assist the person until they receive appropriate professional help or the crisis resolves.

Glossary

Terms are followed by the number of the chapter in which they first appear.

12-step program (8) In a 12-step program, an individual follows an ordered list of increasingly challenging tasks that take him or her along the road of recovery from substance use. In these programs, someone who has completed the 12 steps often guides a newcomer just beginning the steps through the program. Alcoholics Anonymous is the original 12-step program that forms the basis for similar substance use treatment programs.

A

Acceptance and commitment therapy (8) A form of counseling or psychotherapy that uses acceptance and mindfulness strategies that encourage one to open up to unpleasant feelings, to learn how not to overreact to them, and to not avoid situations where such feelings might come up.

Acetylcholine (7) Acetylcholine is a neurotransmitter in the brain. Some antipsychotic medicines bind to acetylcholine receptors in the brain, which may lead to some side effects, like dry mouth, constipation, and blurry vision.

Activity groups (8) Activity groups are a type of group therapy that are based on structured activities. Thus, the focus is less on learning or counseling and more on experiences and activities. These groups work on developing social skills, confidence, and, in some cases, job-related skills.

Acute phase (1) The second of three phases of psychosis, the acute phase is the time during the psychotic episode when symptoms are most disruptive. The acute phase usually lasts until treatment is sought and symptoms are first evaluated and treated.

Adverse events (7) Adverse events are similar to side effects in that they are unwanted effects of medicines, but they are much rarer, may happen at any time when taking the medicine, and sometimes may not go away. Also, adverse events are more serious and at times may even be life-threatening. A serious allergic reaction is an example of an adverse event.

Age of onset (1) The age of onset is the age that psychosis begins. Although it can happen at any time in life, the onset or beginning of a psychotic episode that is diagnosed as a psychotic disorder is usually in late adolescence or early adulthood. For men, the usual age of onset may be earlier than for women. That is, on average, men who develop a psychotic disorder experience their first psychotic symptoms up to three to five years before women do. For example, the symptoms of schizophrenia usually first become apparent in men between the ages of about 20 and 30, and in women between the ages of about 24 and 34.

Aggression (2) See **hostility**.

Anhedonia (2) Anhedonia is a loss of interest or pleasure. People experiencing this negative symptom may not be able to find pleasure in experiences that they used to enjoy. They also may find that they are unable to fully enjoy fun and pleasant things like going to the movies, enjoying a tasty meal, or taking part in hobbies.

Antidepressants (3) These medicines are used to treat major depression. Like other psychiatric medicines, antidepressants are often combined with one or more forms of psychotherapy.

Antipsychotics (7) Antipsychotics are the main types of medicines used to treat psychosis. These medicines are called *antipsychotics* because they fight against ("anti-") psychotic symptoms.

Anxiety (2) It is common for people experiencing psychosis to be anxious or nervous. One source of anxiety may be delusional thoughts. For example, someone may think that people are following him or her, which would make anyone very anxious. Anxiety may show up in some people as being tense or jittery, worrying that something bad is going to happen, or appearing generally uneasy in most situations.

Anxiety medicines (7) Anxiety medicines are a specific type of psychiatric medicines that may be needed if anxiety symptoms are a problem.

Apathy (2) People with apathy, one of the negative symptoms, tend not to care as deeply about what happens in their life. This may include not being upset about negative life events such as losing a job or failing in school.

Assertive community treatment (ACT) (8) ACT is a psychosocial treatment in which a team of mental health professionals brings treatment opportunities to individuals in their own settings. That is, the treatment team comes to the young person (at home), instead of the young person having to come to the treatment team (in a clinic).

Assisted outpatient treatment (6) See **outpatient commitment**.

Atypical antipsychotics (7) Atypical antipsychotics is the name used for the newer antipsychotics. They are considered "atypical" for many reasons, but mainly because they cause much less of the movement side effects often seen with the older "conventional" antipsychotic medicines. They are also called *second-generation antipsychotics* as they are newer than the older *first-generation antipsychotics*.

Auditory hallucinations (2) Auditory hallucinations occur when someone hears voices, even though no one is speaking. These hallucinations may be voices calling one's name, commenting on one's actions, making harsh comments, or giving commands. Individuals with psychosis may react to the voices they are hearing—such as by talking to oneself, whispering to oneself, or looking around as if someone else is talking. The voices are not made up or imagined; the person who hears them is actually hearing the voice because of an abnormality in the brain.

B

Bipolar disorder (3) A mental health professional gives this diagnosis when someone has had one or more episodes of mania. Episodes of major depression may happen in between the episodes of mania. Symptoms of mania may include thinking too highly of oneself (an inflated self-esteem, also called *grandiosity*), not needing to sleep due to having enough energy without sleep, being more talkative than usual, talking very rapidly, having racing thoughts, having poor attention, being agitated, engaging in many different activities, or going on spending sprees. Many cases of mania do not cause psychotic symptoms. However, when the manic episode is severe, psychotic symptoms like hallucinations or delusions may develop.

Blunted affect (2) People with blunted affect show less outward emotion than normal. This negative symptom is observed as decreased facial expression, less use of body language, and a dull tone of voice. A flat affect is a more serious loss of outward emotion, worse than blunted affect.

Brief, intermittent hallucinations (10) Like perceptual abnormalities, brief, intermittent hallucinations may be an early warning sign that hallucinations are about to develop again. Examples of brief, intermittent hallucinations include hearing one's name called out loud that no one else hears or seeing an object or person for a few seconds that no one else sees. Unlike a full hallucination that occurs with psychosis, a brief, intermittent hallucination happens only occasionally and lasts only a few seconds to several minutes.

Brief psychotic disorder (3) People diagnosed with brief psychotic disorder have one or more positive symptoms (hallucinations or delusions) or disorganized speech or behavior, but these symptoms last only up to one month. Functioning then returns to normal and symptoms go away. Brief psychotic disorder may sometimes happen after a very stressful event, such as exposure to a serious natural disaster or being in war or combat.

C

Case management (5) Case management is a service in which one person is in charge of checking in with the individual on a regular basis and making sure that he or she has all the services needed. Case managers are usually nurses, social workers, or other health professionals who help people to coordinate the different parts of their treatment.

Catatonia (2) Catatonia is a rare syndrome that can happen together with the syndrome of psychosis. It is a severe change from normal body movements that happens without a clear reason. For example, those who have catatonia may lose the ability to move, appearing frozen, stiff, and motionless. They also may appear completely unresponsive to their environment. People with psychosis may experience less extreme movement symptoms such as moving very slowly or maintaining unnatural poses.

Civil commitment (6) See **involuntary inpatient treatment.**

Cognitive-behavioral therapy (CBT) (8) CBT is a type of therapy sometimes used for people experiencing an episode of psychosis that targets the specific thoughts and beliefs that an individual has that could make symptoms worse.

Cognitive dysfunction (2) Cognitive dysfunction refers to symptoms that cause difficulties with some of the most important mental functions, like concentration, learning, memory, and planning. Although people with psychosis typically have normal or close to normal intelligence or IQ, they may have some problems with specific cognitive abilities, like the ability to understand, process, and recall information.

Cognitive remediation (8) Cognitive remediation, which may use computerized games and exercises, can be helpful in improving cognitive performance, including difficulties with attention, learning, memory, and planning.

Cognitive tests (2) Psychologists and other mental health professionals assess for cognitive dysfunction using a group of cognitive tests, also referred to as **neurocognitive tests**, or **neuropsychological tests**. Such tests might include giving the meaning of metaphors, having to follow a series of numbers or letters on a computer screen, having to spell things backward, addition and subtraction, seeing how well things are remembered after several minutes have passed, listing as many animals as possible in a one-minute period, completing a series of mazes, and similar tests. Although some of the tests can get difficult, they are often interesting to take part in if one has motivation to do so.

Collateral information (5) Collateral information is additional information gathered by mental health professionals that may confirm the patient's history or provide another perspective on recent problems. Mental health professionals want this information to get several views on what has been going on.

Command hallucinations (2) A form of auditory hallucinations (hearing voices) in which one is told or instructed to do something.

Compulsory treatment (6) See **involuntary inpatient treatment**.

Computerized axial tomography (CAT) scan (6) A CAT scan is commonly used as part of the initial evaluation for psychosis. It is similar to a very detailed X-ray of the brain. It is also known as a **computerized tomography (CT) scan**.

Computerized tomography (CT) scan (6) See **computerized axial tomography (CT) scan**.

Conventional antipsychotics (7) This name is used for the older types of antipsychotics. They are also called *first-generation antipsychotics*. The newer antipsychotics are often referred to as atypical antipsychotics (or *second-generation antipsychotics*).

Co-occurring disorder (8) A co-occurring disorder, also called *comorbidity* or *dual diagnosis*, means that two illnesses are present at the same time. In the context of psychosis, these terms often mean that psychosis occurs at the same time as a substance use disorder.

Coordinated specialty care (5) These are specialty mental health programs that are recovery-oriented and provide treatments proven to be effective for early psychosis. The team of specialists offers medication management geared toward individuals with a first episode of psychosis, using the lowest dose possible. The team also provides psychosocial treatments, including individual psychotherapy, family psychoeducation and support, case management, help with work or school in the form of supported employment and supported education, and other treatments. Following the principles of shared decision-making, both the young person and their family have a voice in treatment decisions based on all of the available options.

Coping (14) Coping means facing and dealing with responsibilities, problems, or difficulties in a successful and healthy way.

D

Day/night reversal (10) Unlike insomnia or hypersomnia, people with day/night reversal get the same amount of sleep as usual but tend to stay awake at night and sleep during the day.

Day treatment programs (8) Day treatment programs are outpatient treatment facilities that provide daytime (but not overnight) treatment to individuals diagnosed with psychosis and other mental illnesses. Both day treatment and partial hospitalization provide a more intensive form of treatment than usual outpatient clinic appointments, without requiring overnight hospital stays.

Delirium (3) Delirium is a state of confusion that develops rapidly, over the course of hours or days. It is usually due to a medical condition, drug use, or withdrawing from certain drugs. Unlike psychosis, delirium often causes disorientation. In addition to causing confusion, delirium can sometimes cause psychotic symptoms, like hallucinations.

Delusional disorder (3) Delusional disorder is similar to schizophrenia, except the main symptom is a single delusion. Delusional disorder is quite rare, but when it does happen, it tends to be somewhat less severe than schizophrenia or schizoaffective disorder because many of the other types of symptoms that may occur with schizophrenia or schizoaffective disorder (like hallucinations, disorganized thinking, negative symptoms, and cognitive dysfunction) are not present.

Delusion of control (2) A delusion of control is the false belief that some other person or an outside force controls one's thoughts, feelings, or actions. For example, a person may be convinced that someone else is putting thoughts into his or her mind through a hex, a curse, or some other means.

Delusions (2) A delusion is a false belief that lasts for a long time. Like hallucinations, delusions are a form of so-called positive symptoms of schizophrenia and related psychotic disorders.

Dementia (3) Dementia causes confusion and disorientation, developing slowly over the course of months or years. Dementia usually occurs in older people, typically after the age of 65 years, and often after the age of 80 years. The most common form of dementia is Alzheimer's disease. In addition to causing confusion, dementia can sometimes cause psychotic symptoms, like hallucinations or delusions.

Depression (3) See **major depression**.

Derailment (2) See **loosening of associations**.

Deterioration in role functioning (10) A deterioration in role functioning is said to occur when people become less able to carry out daily activities and responsibilities. These activities can include work, school, family responsibilities, household chores, personal hygiene, recreation, and socializing. For example, there could be a drop in grades or less social interaction. Or other people might begin to notice poor hygiene. An employer may express concern that one no longer seems to be working as hard as he or she used to.

Diagnosis (2) A diagnosis (plural: diagnoses) is the specific medical term given to an illness or syndrome by healthcare providers.

Diagnostic and Statistical Manual of Mental Disorders (DSM) (3) This book is published by the American Psychiatric Association and is used by mental health professionals in making a psychiatric diagnosis. Another classification of mental illnesses is the **International Classification of Diseases**.

Diathesis–stress model (1) In the diathesis–stress model, it is thought that some people are born with genes that put them at greater risk for having psychosis. However, according to this model, it is thought that genes alone may not be enough to start a psychotic episode.: There must also be a stressor to trigger an episode, such as a stressful life event or drug use. The combination of certain genes and a stressor can cause psychosis.

Differential diagnosis (3) While gathering information to evaluate symptoms of an illness, healthcare providers often come up with a differential diagnosis, or a list of the most likely reasons for the symptoms or syndrome. Healthcare providers generally use a differential diagnosis to list the possible illnesses underlying any health problem. To narrow down this list to the most likely diagnosis, the healthcare provider then uses information from the history (asking questions), physical exam, and lab tests.

Difficulties with abstract thinking (2) In this type of cognitive dysfunction, people with psychosis may not be able to understand complex concepts or solve problems that require them to think through several steps. In addition, they may find it difficult to understand ideas with abstract meanings, such as metaphors, proverbs, and sayings. For example, they may not understand common phrases, like "don't judge a book by its cover" or "there's no use crying over spilled milk."

Difficulties with planning (2) In this type of cognitive dysfunction, people with psychosis may have difficulty making and following through with plans. People may have trouble focusing on future events in a logical way. They also may not have the ability to correctly judge different plans of action. In addition, they may become uncertain and have difficulty making a decision or committing to a plan.

Disorganization (2) Sometimes in psychosis, there are signs of disorganization of thoughts and speech. The normal flow of thinking and speaking can become out of order, confusing, or jumbled. Two examples of disorganization of thoughts are tangentiality and loosening of associations.

Disorganized behavior (2) In addition to the several types of disorganized thoughts and speech, individuals with psychosis may also have disorganized behavior, which often appears as an inability to follow through with plans. It may also be seen in a bizarre appearance, such as having shoes on the wrong feet or wearing clothes inside out. People may dress inappropriately for the weather, wearing several layers of clothing even in warm temperatures. Behavior may also become disorganized because one's thoughts are disorganized.

Disorientation (3) Not knowing the time, place, or situation. This form of confusion can be seen in people with delirium and dementia.

Dopamine (4) Dopamine is a neurotransmitter, a natural chemical in the brain that allows certain neurons to communicate with one another. Psychosis may be caused by a dysfunction in some dopamine pathways.

Drug-induced psychosis (1) Drug-induced psychosis may happen when a person is using drugs like cocaine, LSD, marijuana, methamphetamine, PCP, or synthetic cannabinoids.

Dysphoria (10) Dysphoria is another word for sadness.

E

Early intervention services (5) Specialty clinics that are specifically devoted to people with the early stages of psychosis. In some settings, such services are also called *coordinated specialty care programs.*

Early warning signs (10) Mild symptoms that may occur before the first episode of psychosis and also before later episodes. That is, some mild symptoms may occur during the prodromal phase of the illness, before psychotic symptoms first develop. These same symptoms often serve as warning signs before another episode of illness, or a relapse of psychosis, occurs.

Electroencephalogram (EEG) (6) An EEG records the electrical activity in the brain. To do an EEG, the clinician will attach a number of small electrodes and wires to the person's scalp. The EEG is painless and is commonly used to assess for seizures. Mental health professionals mainly request an EEG to rule out rare seizure disorders, like temporal lobe epilepsy, that sometimes cause psychotic symptoms.

Emotional withdrawal (2) People with emotional withdrawal lack emotional closeness to others. They do not feel like they belong or connect with others, even when spending time with other people. Emotional withdrawal is one of the negative symptoms of schizophrenia and related psychotic disorders.

Extrapyramidal side effects (EPS or EPSE) (7) EPS are a number of movement side effects, which can be quite common when taking conventional antipsychotics. They are less likely to occur when taking the newer atypical antipsychotic medicines. They include acute dystonia, akathisia, and parkinsonism.

F

Family interventions (8) There are several forms of family interventions, all of which focus on helping the family as a whole rather than just the young person. Such interventions view each member of the family as having an important role or purpose. Without that member's involvement in the family system, the system would not work as well.

Family psychoeducation (8) Like individual psychoeducation or psychoeducational groups for young people with psychosis themselves, family psychoeducation teaches family members about symptoms, diagnoses, evaluations, treatments, and other topics relevant to psychosis. Additionally, and perhaps most importantly, family members learn to recognize the symptoms of a relapse (early warning signs) and strategies for reducing the chance of future relapses.

Family therapy (8) Family therapy is a form of family intervention that may be helpful in reducing the chance of relapse or rehospitalization after a first episode. This is because family therapy directly targets stressors in the young person's immediate environment. Because family stress may worsen the symptoms of someone in the early stages of psychosis, possibly leading to a relapse, family therapy focuses on improving communication and problem-solving skills. It strengthens the family's best coping skills, while minimizing challenges and interaction styles that could create stress.

Fasting glucose and lipids (7) Because of the possibility of some side effects, doctors prescribing antipsychotics closely monitor the patient's weight and periodically check certain labs, like fasting glucose (sugar) and lipids. This requires drawing a sample of blood to be sent to the lab.

First-episode psychosis (1) First-episode psychosis is the period of time when a person first begins to experience psychosis.

Flat affect (2) A flat affect is a loss of outward emotion, worse than blunted affect. People with this negative symptom have an almost complete absence of facial expressions and body language, resulting in a very dull appearance and tone of voice.

G

Generic name (7) A generic name is one of two names of a medicine. For example, acetaminophen is the generic name for Tylenol.

Genes (4) Genes are segments of DNA that pass along the "blueprints" of how the body's cells are to make proteins.

Glutamate (4) Glutamate is a neurotransmitter, a natural chemical in the brain that allows certain neurons to communicate with one another. Psychosis may be caused by a dysfunction in some glutamate pathways.

Grandiose delusion (2) A grandiose delusion is the false belief that one has high social status, is famous, has large amounts of money, or has special powers.

Group therapy (8) Group therapy is a psychosocial treatment in which one or two mental health professionals lead a group of people in a discussion or a planned activity. It allows young people to learn not only from the therapist, but also from the interactions between the therapist and other group members, and the interactions between group members themselves.

H

Hallucinations (2) A hallucination is a false experience of one of the five senses (hearing, seeing, feeling, smelling, and tasting). Even though hallucinations may happen in any of the five senses, auditory hallucinations (hearing voices) are the most common. Like delusions, hallucinations are a type of the so-called positive symptoms of schizophrenia and related psychotic disorders.

Heritable (4) Heritable means that an illness is partly caused by genes. Many illnesses that are associated with psychosis, like schizophrenia, are heritable, or partly caused by genes, even though they may not appear to run in families.

Histamine (7) Histamine is a neurotransmitter in the brain. Some antipsychotics may bind to histamine receptors in the brain, which may lead to side effects like sleepiness.

Hostility (2) Most people experiencing psychosis are not dangerous or violent in any way, and the rate of violence in people experiencing psychosis is very similar to that of the population as a whole. However, some people with psychosis do show increased hostility or **aggression**. They may argue more than normal, destroy property, or make threats toward others. Although rare, when these behaviors do occur, they can be driven by specific delusions. For example, someone with a paranoid delusion may act out of fear, believing that they must do something for protection and safety.

Hypersomnia (10) Hypersomnia means sleeping more than usual. It can be seen as the opposite of **insomnia**.

I

Ideas of reference (2) Ideas of reference are when one believes that others are talking about them or that things are referring especially to them when they really are not. For example, someone might believe that the television or radio newscasters are talking about them or are trying to send coded messages. This might prompt the person to remove or even destroy the television or radio because of these troubling false ideas.

Imaging studies (6) See **neuroimaging**.

Impaired information processing (2) In this type of cognitive dysfunction, people experiencing this symptom may have difficulty sorting out information and discovering meaning in things that they observe. It may appear that things do not "sink in" the way they used to or that complex concepts seem more difficult for them to understand than before.

Impaired insight (2) Impaired insight (often referred to as **unawareness of illness**) is a common experience for people with psychosis. Because their unusual experiences may be very real to them, people experiencing psychosis do not realize that the thoughts and behaviors they are having are a change from their normal self. They also may be unaware that their behavior is different from that of other people. People with impaired insight might refuse to take medicines or follow up with treatment because they simply don't see or recognize a need for it.

Individual Placement and Support (IPS) (13) A model of support for employment goals (or school goals) that is often a part of treatment programs for individuals with serious mental illnesses. Some of its principles include zero exclusion (meaning that anyone interested in getting a job is eligible for services), rapid engagement and employment, a focus on competitive (meaning paid rather than volunteer) employment, being integrated with the rest of the treatment team, continuing support after getting a job, and valuing clients' own preferences. IPS is the main model of supported employment, which is a psychosocial treatment that focuses on work goals.

Individualized Education Plan (IEP) (13) A plan developed in elementary, middle, and high schools for a student with a disability to ensure they are receiving the additional supports necessary for academic success.

Insomnia (10) Insomnia is a difficulty in falling asleep or staying asleep. For example, insomnia may mean taking more than 30 minutes to fall asleep or waking up in the middle of the night and not being able to go back to sleep. It can also be waking up more than 30 minutes earlier than one wanted in the morning.

Integrated treatment programs (8) Mental health professionals in these programs focus on both the treatment of psychosis and substance use at the same time in the same setting.

International Classification of Diseases (ICD) (3) This classification used by mental health professionals provides specific definitions of psychiatric disorders and is produced by the World Health Organization. Another classification of mental illnesses is the *Diagnostic and Statistical Manual of Mental Disorders* (DSM), produced by the American Psychiatric Association.

Involuntary community treatment (6) See **outpatient commitment**.

Involuntary hospitalization (6) See **involuntary inpatient treatment**.

Involuntary inpatient treatment (6) In involuntary inpatient treatment, the patient has symptoms that require hospitalization, but he or she does not agree to sign in to the hospital. A psychiatrist can then keep the young person in the hospital, depending on state/provincial or national laws. This is also called *involuntary hospitalization, civil commitment*, or *compulsory treatment*.

L

Life events (14) Life events are one kind of stressor and include things such as becoming ill, experiencing the death of a loved one, going through a divorce, getting married, having a baby, getting a new job, or moving. Some life events are more stressful than others.

Loosening of associations (2) Unlike tangentiality, which is a similar form of disorganization, loosening of associations (also called **derailment**) is when one idea does not match the next at all. The ideas do not connect in any logical way. Ideas shift from one subject to another in a completely unrelated way. The thinking process is "loose" instead of being tightly ordered and logical.

Low drive, energy, or motivation (2) Young people experiencing this negative symptom may have lost the desire to finish school, to be in a relationship, to get a job, or to participate in social activities.

Lumbar puncture (6) This medical procedure is performed by doctors to rule out an infection in the brain by examining cerebrospinal fluid. Such tests may also need to be done to rule out any potential inflammatory process that causes encephalopathy (brain inflammation), which can bring about psychotic symptoms. It is also known as a **spinal tap**.

M

Magnetic resonance imaging (MRI) (6) An imaging study, or form of neuroimaging, that allows mental health professionals to see any abnormalities, such as tumors, swelling inside the brain, or small areas of disease that might cause psychotic symptoms. The MRI uses magnetic waves instead of X-ray radiation.

Major depression (3) Also called *major depressive disorder* or *clinical depression*, this is when one has been experiencing multiple symptoms of depression for at least two weeks. A depressive episode may last weeks, months, or even years. Symptoms may include feeling sad or depressed, not being as interested in fun or pleasurable things, a decreased or increased appetite, weight loss or weight gain, having difficulty sleeping, sleeping too much, feeling agitated, feeling slow, fatigue, loss of energy, feeling worthless, feeling guilty for no apparent reason, having difficulty concentrating or making decisions, or having thoughts of death or thoughts of committing suicide. Major depression is a common psychiatric disorder—much more common than schizophrenia and other primary psychotic disorders. In most cases, major depression does not cause psychosis. However, in some instances, when the depression becomes severe, psychotic symptoms may develop (this is sometimes called *psychotic depression*).

Mania (3) Mania is an episode of abnormally elevated or excited mood, such as periods in which the person feels abnormally good, high, or excited. Symptoms may include thinking too highly of oneself (an inflated self-esteem, also called *grandiosity*), not needing to sleep due to having enough energy without sleep, being more talkative than usual, talking very rapidly, having racing thoughts, having poor attention, being agitated, engaging in many different activities, or going on spending sprees. People who have a manic episode often receive a diagnosis of bipolar disorder or schizoaffective disorder—bipolar type.

Mental illness (1) A mental illness is a health condition that affects a person's thoughts, feelings, and behaviors. Like physical illnesses, mental illnesses are treatable.

Mental status exam (6) A mental status exam is part of the interview done by a mental health professional during an evaluation. The mental status exam includes an assessment of several aspects of mental functioning, including appearance, attitude, behavior, speech, mood, affect, thought process, thought content, insight, judgment, impulse control, and cognition.

Metabolic side effects (7) Antipsychotic medicines can sometimes cause metabolic side effects, which include elevations in blood sugar and cholesterol levels. Doctors monitor for these side effects because they can have negative effects on long-term health.

Mobile crisis teams (6) Sometimes an initial or follow-up evaluation has to be done at home, especially if the person refuses to go to see a mental health professional. In some cases, this evaluation might be done by a mobile crisis team, which usually includes two or three people who go to talk with someone who may have a mental health condition in his or her home, school, or wherever else he or she might be.

Mood stabilizers (3) These medicines are used to treat bipolar disorder, often in combination with certain types of psychotherapy. They may also be useful if irritability, impulsiveness, hostility, or unstable moods are present even if bipolar disorder is not the diagnosis.

Motivational enhancement therapy (11) A form of counseling or therapy that aims to increase one's desire or motivation to quit smoking (or change some other behavior) over the course of several sessions with a mental health professional. **Motivational interviewing** is a very similar type of counseling.

Motivational interviewing (11) See **motivational enhancement therapy**.

Multi-family groups (8) Family psychoeducation may take place within a single family or within multi-family groups, in which family members from several different families that are going through the same thing are present. Multi-family groups can be helpful because family members can talk to and learn from other families who also have a loved one experiencing psychosis.

N

Negative symptoms (2) Negative symptoms are a group of symptoms of psychosis in which things that people should normally do or think are now missing. In other words, these symptoms have *subtracted*, or removed, something from their experience (which is why they are called *negative symptoms*). Some negative symptoms include anhedonia; apathy; blunted affect or flat affect; emotional withdrawal; low drive, energy, or motivation; poor attention to grooming and hygiene; slow or empty thinking and speech; slow movements; and social isolation.

Neurocognitive tests (2) See **cognitive tests.**

Neurodevelopmental model (1) The neurodevelopmental model posits that psychosis is the result of minor injuries to the brain during its growth and development or biological mishaps during brain development.

Neuroimaging (6) Neuroimaging allow radiologists and mental health professionals to look at the brain to determine if there are any abnormal findings, such as brain tumors or evidence of infections. These medical procedures are also called **imaging studies.**

Neurons (4) Neurons are cells in the brain.

Neuropsychological tests (2) See **cognitive tests.**

Neurotransmitters (4) The substances needed for communication between neurons in the brain. Examples include dopamine and glutamate.

Nicotine replacement therapy (11) Nicotine replacement therapy can be very helpful for someone trying to stop smoking. Smoking cessation programs typically offer nicotine replacement in the form of a gum, patch, lozenge, inhaler, or nasal spray. These non-dangerous substitutes for nicotine make it easier to reduce or quit smoking.

Norepinephrine (7) Norepinephrine is a neurotransmitter in the brain. Some antipsychotics may bind to norepinephrine receptors, and this may cause certain side effects, like low blood pressure.

O

Ongoing stressors (14) Ongoing stressors are a part of everyone's life. Some of these include unwanted or unpleasant household chores, frequent or repeated arguments or conflicts, financial problems, constant criticism, being unemployed, or a chronic illness in a loved one.

Open Dialogue (8) This treatment model is a person-centered approach that builds on the strengths of the individual at the center of concern and promotes shared decision-making. It can be used to help people plan their treatment, if they are in crisis, or to support an individual and their family in an ongoing way. Open Dialogue treatment is carried out through network meetings involving the young person and his or her family members and social network, along with at least two mental health professionals.

Other specified schizophrenia spectrum and other psychotic disorder (3) Although the name of this diagnosis is confusing, it means that the symptoms of a primary psychotic disorder (like schizophrenia) are present, but the "full criteria" for any of the five psychotic disorders are not met. Mental health professionals making this diagnosis can then "specify" further what is meant.

Outpatient commitment (6) A court order may be used to ensure that the patient stays in outpatient treatment. If he or she fails to continue outpatient treatment, then hospitalization may be necessary. Outpatient commitment is also called **involuntary community treatment** or **assisted outpatient treatment.**

Overvalued ideas (10) An overvalued idea is when too much emphasis is placed on an idea. Overvalued ideas can involve religious or philosophical thoughts, wondering about the ability to read others' minds, believing too much in superstitions, or other ideas that one is overly concerned with.

P

Paranoia (2) See **suspiciousness.**

Paranoid delusion (2) A paranoid delusion is the false belief that one is being plotted against or followed. For example, a person may believe that the FBI has planted a camera in the walls and his or her family is part of a government plot.

Partial hospitalization programs (8) Partial hospitalization programs are outpatient treatment programs that provide daytime (but not overnight) treatment to individuals diagnosed with psychosis and other mental illnesses. Partial hospitalization, like day treatment, provides a more intensive form of treatment than usual outpatient clinic appointments, without requiring overnight hospital stays.

Peer specialists (5) Peer specialists are individuals who themselves have gone through evaluation and treatment for a mental illness like a psychotic disorder, and who now have a job as part of the mental health team. They have a special role in assisting young people with psychosis and their family members because they have the "lived experience" of what it's like to be in treatment and to be engaged in recovery. Peer specialists are also sometimes called *peer counselors* or *peer navigators*.

Peer support (12) Counseling and support from peer specialists who work as part of the mental health treatment team.

Perceptual abnormality (10) A perceptual abnormality is when the experience of one of the five senses (hearing, seeing, feeling, tasting, or smelling) changes enough that the person wonders if their mind might be playing tricks on them. Examples include mistaking a noise for voices whispering, hearing one's name called in a noisy room, briefly seeing someone else's face when looking in a mirror, seeing something out of the corner of one's eye incorrectly, or thinking that a spot on the wall at first glance looks like an object of some sort.

Poor attention and concentration (2) In this type of cognitive dysfunction, people experiencing psychosis often display limitations in attention and concentration. They may have a hard time keeping their thoughts on one idea. They also may find tasks that require them to focus their attention to be very tiring. For example, they may find it difficult to stay focused on a book or a television show for more than a few minutes.

Poor attention to grooming and hygiene (2) Poor attention to grooming and hygiene can include not bathing, not brushing one's teeth, wearing dirty clothes, or not combing one's hair. This neglect can happen for many reasons; for example, it may be the result of other negative symptoms, like apathy and low motivation.

Poor memory (2) In this type of cognitive dysfunction, people experiencing poor memory usually have trouble learning and remembering new things. Some also may have trouble remembering past events, but this is much less common.

Positive symptoms (2) The most outwardly obvious symptoms of psychosis are positive symptoms. The use of the word *positive* is often confusing; it does not mean that these symptoms are enjoyable or helpful. They are things that young people should not normally do or think. In other words, these symptoms are abnormal experiences *added* *on* (which is why they are called *positive*) to normal psychological experience. Positive symptoms include hallucinations, delusions, suspiciousness/paranoia, and ideas of reference.

Postpartum psychosis (3) Postpartum psychosis is diagnosed when a woman has psychotic symptoms anytime within the first three months after giving birth. The symptoms usually begin within the first month after the child's birth and usually come on fairly suddenly. Unlike postpartum depression, which involves depressive symptoms, postpartum psychosis involves having psychotic symptoms, like hallucinations or delusions. Postpartum psychosis usually gets better with treatment.

Poverty of content of speech (2) This means that what one is talking about may seem unclear, meaningless, or vague. For example, a person may have the same answer for every question asked, or have very little to say. This form of disorganization is similar to the negative symptom of slow or empty thinking and speech.

Primary psychotic disorders (3) A group of psychiatric disorders that cause psychosis. They are called this because they primarily cause psychosis, rather than depression, anxiety, or another type of syndrome. The most common of these is schizophrenia, followed by other disorders closely related to schizophrenia.

Prodromal phase (1) As the first of three phases of psychosis, the prodromal phase is the time before a psychotic episode begins, when subtle symptoms may first appear. The prodromal phase may last from several weeks to several years. It is often not recognized as the early stages of a mental illness.

Prodromal symptoms (1) Prodromal symptoms are subtle changes in thoughts, feelings, or behaviors that may have occurred before the first episode of psychosis began. Family and friends may have noticed these changes. They may see changes in mood, sleep habits, and participation in social activities. These same mild symptoms may occur again before another episode of psychosis. Some people with psychosis may not have had any prodromal symptoms at all.

Prolactin (7) Prolactin is a hormone secreted by the pituitary gland in the brain. When taking conventional antipsychotics, and some atypical antipsychotics, the prolactin level in the blood may rise. This may cause some side effects.

Psychiatric advance directive (15) A set of instructions that a person would like followed if a relapse of illness occurs. It is a legal document written by a currently competent person who has a mental illness. It allows a person to be prepared if a mental health crisis prevents them from being able to make decisions. A psychiatric advance directive describes treatment preferences, or names a person to make treatment decisions, should the person with a mental illness be unable to make decisions.

Psychiatrist (6) A psychiatrist is a medical doctor who has received specialty training in psychiatry. Psychiatrists evaluate and treat people with mental illnesses and often prescribe medicines as part of the treatment.

Psychoeducation (8) A type of education that focuses on the topic of mental illnesses. The goal of psychoeducation is to help individuals with a mental illness, and their family members, better understand the illness. If a person understands his or her illness, then he or she will be able to deal with it more successfully. Psychoeducation, for both young people and their families, is an effective form of treatment in itself and an important step in preventing relapse and hospitalization.

Psychoeducational groups (8) These are groups that teach young people about psychosis in a clear, structured way, similar to a small class. In psychoeducational groups, young people learn from mental health professionals about symptoms, treatments, early warning signs, and other topics relevant to psychosis.

Psychologist (6) A psychologist is similar to a psychiatrist but has received training in the field of psychology rather than in medicine. Although psychologists are usually not licensed to prescribe medicines, they have other specialized skills, such as performing formal psychological testing (like cognitive tests).

Psychosis (1) Psychosis is a word used to describe a person's mental state when he or she has in some way become disconnected from reality. For example, a person might hear voices that are not really there (auditory hallucinations) or believe things that are not really true (delusions). Psychosis is a treatable medical condition that occurs due to a dysfunction in the brain.

Psychosis continuum (1) This phrase is used to describe the different levels of psychotic experiences. This means that there is a range of severity or seriousness across the different types of experiences of psychosis. The different types of psychotic experiences range from normal experiences that are similar to psychosis and that cause little or no distress, to the full syndrome of psychosis that causes much distress or many problems in life.

Psychosis-prone (1) Some people are more likely to develop psychotic symptoms than others. They may or may not develop psychosis, but they have a tendency toward it.

Psychosis related to a medical problem (1) People with certain physical illnesses, such as meningitis, certain types of seizures, or a brain tumor, may experience psychosis related to a medical problem.

Psychosocial development (8) Psychosocial development refers to the important developmental stage when psychological and social skills mature. It begins in childhood and continues throughout adolescence and early adulthood. Adolescence and early adulthood are very important times when people develop social skills and build relationships. This period is typically a time of finishing high school, starting college, getting a first job, having a first romantic relationship, beginning to live more independently from one's parents, getting one's first car, and establishing career goals.

Psychosocial rehabilitation (8) This term is sometimes used to describe many psychosocial treatments. This means that treatment improves a person's psychosocial skills so that the individual can function at the best possible level. In other words, psychosocial rehabilitation aims to reduce challenges and maximize abilities in areas such as school, work, relationships, and recreation/leisure.

Psychosocial treatments (5) They are called *psychosocial* treatments because they address both psychological problems (like the symptoms of psychosis) and social problems (like needing to get back to school or work). These treatments aim to help the person with symptoms of psychosis and with other problems that sometimes occur as a result of psychosis. Psychosocial treatments may focus on depression, substance abuse, getting back to school or work, and improving relationships. Psychosocial treatments are very helpful, especially in combination with medicines, for people who are moving toward recovery. Psychosocial treatments often include individual therapy sessions, classes, or group sessions.

Psychotic (1) This word describes someone who is experiencing psychosis, having either hallucinations or delusions.

Psychotic disorder (1) A psychotic disorder is a mental illness that brings about psychosis that interferes with life. Some people with a psychotic disorder have repeating episodes but are able to function normally between these episodes. Others may have repeating psychotic episodes without a full recovery between them. Yet others may have only one psychotic episode in their lifetime.

Psychotic episode (1) A psychotic episode is a period of time during which someone has psychotic symptoms. These symptoms may make it difficult for the person to carry out daily activities. A psychotic episode may last from days to weeks, or in some cases even months or years, depending on the person and the treatments received.

R

Receptors (7) Receptors are proteins on the surface of cells, such as nerve cells or neurons. Medicines bind to receptors once they are in the brain.

Recovery (12) Recovery means successfully living with a mental illness by not being confined by it; embracing hope, empowerment, and self-determination; and focusing on one's personal life goals and roles in society. It differs from remission because it focuses on more than just symptom control. Instead, recovery focuses on personal goals decided by individuals themselves. Some basic principles of recovery are that there are many pathways to recovery, it is self-directed and empowering, it requires a personal recognition of the need for change, it is holistic and strengths-based, it considers cultural backgrounds, and it involves whole health and wellness.

Recovery model (3) The recovery model of mental health treatment aims to empower the individual to achieve his or her own goals for treatment and recovery by actively participating in treatment decisions.

Recovery phase (1) The third of three phases of psychosis, the recovery phase is the time after the psychotic episode when symptoms of psychosis lessen or sometimes go away completely with treatment. The recovery phase is often considered to be the first six to 18 months of treatment.

Referral (8) A referral is when a healthcare professional recommends that a person goes to a particular type of treatment.

Relapse (2) A relapse is when psychotic symptoms reappear and there is a worsening or return of illness.

Relapse prevention (10) The goal of preventing a relapse (or recurrence of symptoms), by sticking with treatment, watching for early warning signs, and intervening promptly.

Religious delusion (2) A religious delusion is the false belief that one has religious importance, such as being a biblical figure.

Remission (7) Remission means that the major symptoms, usually positive symptoms like hallucinations and delusions, are no longer active. The goals of remission and recovery go hand in hand. But recovery is a much broader concept, pertaining to one's life goals, rather than to just getting symptoms under control.

Risk factors (4) A risk factor is any event or exposure that occurs before the illness and that research has shown plays a role in causing the illness. Research has identified a number of risk factors for psychosis.

Risk genes (4) Risk genes are genes that each play a small role in a person's likelihood of developing an illness, like psychosis.

S

Schizoaffective disorder (3) People with schizoaffective disorder have a combination of psychotic symptoms and serious mood symptoms. The mood symptoms may be like the symptoms seen in clinical depression, also called major depression, or they may be like the symptoms seen in mania, or bipolar disorder. So, there are two types of schizoaffective disorder.

Schizoaffective disorder—bipolar type (3) People diagnosed with schizoaffective disorder—bipolar type have the symptoms of schizophrenia, but also at times have symptoms of **mania**. These may include thinking too highly of oneself (an inflated self-esteem, also called grandiosity), not needing to sleep due to having enough energy without sleep, being more talkative than usual, talking very rapidly, having racing thoughts, having poor attention, being agitated, engaging in many different activities, or going on spending sprees.

Schizoaffective disorder—depressive type (3) People diagnosed with schizoaffective disorder—depressive type have the symptoms of schizophrenia, but also at times have symptoms of depression. These may include feeling sad or depressed, not being as interested in fun or pleasurable things, a decreased or increased appetite, weight loss or weight gain, having difficulty sleeping or sleeping too much, feeling agitated, feeling slow, fatigue, loss of energy, feeling worthless, feeling guilty for no apparent reason, having difficulty concentrating or making decisions, or having thoughts of death or thoughts of committing suicide.

Schizophrenia (3) People with schizophrenia have a combination of psychotic symptoms. Specifically, schizophrenia is defined by the presence of two or more of the following: delusions, hallucinations, disorganized speech, disorganized or catatonic behavior, and negative symptoms, and the illness lasts for longer than six months. So, schizophrenia is very similar to schizophreniform disorder except that in schizophrenia, symptoms last longer. In fact, schizophrenia usually lasts for a very long time and may even be lifelong.

Schizophreniform disorder (3) People diagnosed with schizophreniform disorder have a combination of psychotic symptoms that last at least one month, and up to six months. The combination of symptoms includes two or more of the following: delusions, hallucinations, disorganized speech, disorganized or catatonic behavior, and negative symptoms. Schizophreniform disorder is a psychotic episode that lasts longer than brief psychotic disorder, but does not last long enough to receive a diagnosis of schizophrenia. If the symptoms last for longer than six months, then the diagnosis is changed from schizophreniform disorder to schizophrenia or one of the other primary psychotic disorders.

Schizotypal disorder (1) See **schizotypal personality disorder**.

Schizotypal personality disorder (1) When many schizotypal personality features are present and long-lasting, a person might be diagnosed by mental health professionals as having schizotypal personality disorder (or just **schizotypal disorder**). Schizotypal personality disorder is a stable set of personality traits that appear as a milder form of the symptoms of schizophrenia.

Schizotypal personality features (1) People who experience mild, ongoing difficulties from symptoms but usually still function well enough to work and maintain relationships may have schizotypal personality features. People with schizotypal personality features can seem to have fewer social skills at times or may have suspicious or paranoid thinking. They also tend to withdraw from society. Typically, they do not experience full hallucinations or delusions.

Serotonin (7) Serotonin is a natural chemical in the brain, a neurotransmitter, that plays a role in the mental functions affected by psychosis, anxiety, and depression. Some antipsychotics bind to serotonin receptors, and this may account for some of their beneficial effects.

Severity (1) Severity refers to the levels of seriousness of symptoms and experiences of psychosis.

Shared decision-making (5) An approach to treatment in which both the person receiving treatment and their family have a voice in treatment decisions based on all of the available options. Decisions about treatment are made as a collaborative process.

Side effects (7) Side effects are unwanted effects of medicines.

Signs (2) Signs are like symptoms, but a doctor sees them through an interview, exam, or test. In contrast, symptoms are experienced by the individual, who may not even know that he or she has signs of an illness.

Sleep medicines (7) Sleep medicines are sometimes used to treat insomnia. They may be needed if people with psychosis have difficulty sleeping.

Slow movements (2) Individuals with slow movements as a negative symptom may walk, move, and talk more slowly than normal.

Slow or empty thinking and speech (2) People experiencing this negative symptom may seem like they are unable to keep up with the conversation. There may also be a long period between asking a question and their response to it. It may seem like they have very few thoughts.

Smoking cessation (11) The process of quitting smoking.

Smoking cessation medicines (11) Several smoking cessation medicines, including bupropion (Wellbutrin, Zyban) and varenicline (Chantix), are available to make quitting easier.

Social isolation (2) People experiencing social isolation as a negative symptom may become unconcerned with relationships that had been close and important to them before. They usually have difficulty forming new relationships. They may instead spend most of their time alone.

Social skills (8) Social skills are the daily skills that allow us to successfully interact with one another and have rewarding relationships. Good social skills allow us to have close, supportive relationships with others. Developing psychotic symptoms during late adolescence or early adulthood often disrupts the process of social development and interferes with key social milestones.

Social skills training (8) Social skills training is a psychosocial treatment that helps individuals to improve or regain their prior level of social skills, or to resume development of social skills interrupted by psychosis. Social skills training focuses on teaching people how to approach and navigate personal and professional social situations through a combination of coaching, practicing within the clinic, getting feedback from mental health professionals or peers in the group, and then trying it out in the real world. An important part of social skills training is repetition of the targeted skill.

Social withdrawal (10) People who have social withdrawal are generally not interested in having social contact with others and are less likely to become involved socially. It can appear as if they are pulling back from social situations or that they have poor social skills. Even if they will still join in on social activities when others approach them, they tend to not seek out socializing opportunities themselves.

Somatic delusion (2) A somatic delusion is the false belief that something is wrong with one's body. For example, a person may believe that there is a parasite in his or her skin or that a cancer or tumor is growing in his or her body.

Spinal tap (6) See **lumbar puncture**.

Stigma (12) A society's stereotypes, misbeliefs, and discrimination toward certain groups of people, such as those with a mental illness. Stigma is a form of discrimination that stems from lack of understanding about mental illnesses.

Stress (14) This word describes a feeling of strain, pressure, or tension.

Stressful life events (4) Various stressful life events may be risk factors for schizophrenia or may worsen the symptoms of psychosis. Such difficulties may include child abuse, discrimination, poverty, and the sense of "social defeat" that these problems may lead to.

Stress-induced psychosis (1) People who experience a great deal of physical stress from lack of sleep, hunger, or torture, or severe psychological stress, may experience stress-induced psychosis.

Stressors (14) Stressors are events that cause stress. In general, there are two types of stressors, life events and ongoing stressors.

Substance use disorder (11) People receive a diagnosis of a substance use disorder when the use of a substance interferes with their ability to perform on the job, disrupts relationships, or results in legal problems, among other problems.

Suicidal ideation (2) See **suicidal thoughts**.

Suicidal thoughts (2) People experiencing psychosis may have thoughts about dying. This may include wishing to be dead, as well as thinking about or planning to commit suicide. Suicidal thoughts (also called **suicidal ideation**) may be driven by several symptoms, including emotional distress due to the frightening experience of psychosis or as a direct result of hallucinations or delusions.

Supported education (8) This psychosocial treatment is similar to supported employment, but rather than focusing on assistance with work, it supports young people with first-episode psychosis in late adolescence or early adulthood to complete their education and achieve their educational goals.

Supported employment (8) Supported employment programs help people with serious mental illnesses to work either part time or full time, while keeping their preferences at the forefront. Such programs try to place young people in the type of work that best fits them in terms of interests, skills, and comfort level.

Supportive housing (8) This type of psychosocial treatment provides a safe, supportive place to live for patients with serious mental illnesses.

Supportive psychotherapy (8) A type of counseling or psychotherapy that supports and builds one's best coping skills.

Suspiciousness (2) Suspiciousness or **paranoia** exists when a person with psychosis has the concern that those around them are trying to cause problems in their life. Sometimes suspiciousness may be so severe that it is a **paranoid delusion**. Other suspiciousness may be milder and result in people isolating themselves from others because they do not trust them. People with paranoia may not ask for help because they believe that others are trying to harm them rather than help them.

Symptom (2) A symptom is an obvious change from one's normal health that happens when an illness or disease occurs. Symptoms often are the reason you go to a doctor or other healthcare provider.

Syndrome (2) A combination of both symptoms and signs.

T

Tangentiality (2) Tangentiality is a form of disorganization. It happens when one idea connects to the next, but the thoughts become confusing because they go off on a tangent and end on a different subject. The person starts talking about one topic, but veers off on an unrelated tangent and never gets back to the original topic.

Tardive dyskinesia (TD) (7) TD is an adverse event that develops after extended periods (months, years, or decades) of taking conventional antipsychotics. TD consists of abnormal, involuntary movements. These movements often involve the mouth (chewing or puckering movements), the fingers or toes, or the trunk (such as rocking or swaying).

Therapy groups (8) These groups focus on helping young people explore their relationships, their coping styles, and stressors that may make symptoms worse. Young people work on understanding themselves and the things they do that may interfere with psychosocial success.

Thought blocking (2) Thought blocking is a form of disorganization that happens when there is an interruption in the train of thought and the person cannot put his or her thoughts into words. The thoughts are "blocked" from coming out. So, the person may be very slow to respond to questions or may not be able to respond at all. At other times, rather than actual thought blocking, the person may be too distracted to respond, such as if they are hearing voices and can't pay attention to both the voices and you at the same time.

Trade name (7) A trade name is one of two names of a medicine. For example, Tylenol is a trade name for acetaminophen. All medicines have both a trade name and a generic name.

Treatment-resistant psychosis (7) Patients with treatment-resistant psychosis have psychotic symptoms that have not cleared up even after trying two or more different antipsychotic medicines. Clozapine, one of the atypical antipsychotics, is much more helpful than other medicines for treatment-resistant psychosis.

U

Unawareness of illness (2) See **impaired insight**.

Unspecified schizophrenia spectrum and other psychotic disorder (3) People given this diagnosis have symptoms of a primary psychotic disorder (like schizophrenia) but do not meet "full criteria" for any of the five primary psychotic disorders. Mental health professionals using this diagnosis do not specify further details. This diagnosis is most often used when there is not yet enough information to make one of the five specific diagnoses described earlier. That is, mental health professionals often use this as a preliminary diagnosis before deciding on a more conclusive diagnosis once more information is obtained. Sometimes a person may receive a new, updated diagnosis when more is learned about a person's symptoms and a more detailed evaluation can be conducted.

V

Voluntary hospitalization (6) See **voluntary inpatient treatment**.

Voluntary inpatient treatment (6) In the case of voluntary inpatient treatment, the patient chooses willingly to sign into the hospital. Also known as **voluntary hospitalization**.

W

Weight gain (7) Weight gain is one of the side effects that may happen when taking some antipsychotics.

Working diagnosis (3) The most likely diagnosis given all available information, which is used to guide treatment planning even if a final diagnosis cannot yet be made.

Index

Tables, figures, and boxes are indicated by *t*, *f*, and *b* following the page number.

For the benefit of digital users, indexed terms that span two pages (e.g., 52–53) may, on occasion, appear on only one of those pages.

12-step program, 114, 189

AA (Alcoholics Anonymous), 114, 142
abnormal experiences, 7–8
abnormalities in brain development, 52–53, 54–55, 56f
acceptance and commitment therapy, 109, 189–90
acetylcholine, 86, 189–90
ACT (assertive community treatment), 115, 189–90
activity groups, 110, 189–90
acute phase, 12–13, 189–90
Addison's disease, 37–38
ADHD (attention-deficit/hyperactivity disorder), 39
adolescence. *See* childhood and adolescence
adverse events, 87–88, 189–90
affect, 73
age of onset, 7, 42–43, 189–90
aggression. *See* hostility
alcohol, 139–40
Alcoholics Anonymous (AA), 114, 142
allergic reactions, 90
Alzheimer's disease, 46–47
anhedonia, 22, 189–90
antidepressants, 45, 96, 189–90
antipsychotics, 83–101, 84b
    additional medicines to, 96
    adverse events, 87–88
    atypical, 91–94, 92t
    benefits of, 97b, 97, 98f
    choosing, 94–96
    conventional, 88–91, 89t
    defined, 189–90
    duration of treatment, 98–99
    medicines prescribed worksheet, 100
    movement side effects, 28
    overview, 83–85, 99–101
    relapse prevention and, 135
    side effects, 86–87, 87t
    specialty care programs, 64
    sticking with treatment, 120–121
    substance use with, 140
antisocial personality disorder, 6
anxiety, 28, 189–90
anxiety medicines, 96, 189–90
apathy, 22, 189–90
appearance, 72
aripiprazole, 95
Artane (trihexyphenidyl), 89
assertive community treatment (ACT), 115, 189–90
assisted outpatient treatment. *See* outpatient commitment
Atarax (hydroxyzine), 89
attention, poor, 26–27, 201–5
attention-deficit/hyperactivity disorder (ADHD), 39
attitude, 73
atypical antipsychotics, 91–94, 92t, 189–90
auditory hallucinations, 20, 189–90
autoimmune disorders, 37–38

behavior, 73
Benadryl (diphenhydramine), 89
benztropine (Cogentin), 89
bipolar disorder, 45–46, 191
bizarre delusions, 21
blunted affect, 22, 133, 191
brain development abnormalities, 52–53, 54–55
brain injuries, 12
brief, intermittent hallucinations, 132, 191
brief psychotic disorder, 41, 191
bupropion (Wellbutrin, Zyban), 140–41

case management, 63, 191–93
CAT (computerized axial tomography) scan, 77, 191–93
catatonia, 27–28, 191–93
CBT (cognitive-behavioral therapy), 106–9, 121, 191–93
cerebrospinal fluid, 76
Chantix (varenicline), 140–41
childhood and adolescence, 12, 53–54, 54*f*. *See also* psychosocial treatments
childhood-onset schizophrenia, 42–43
cigarette smoking, 139–40
civil commitment. *See* involuntary inpatient treatment
clozapine (Clozaril), 93–94, 141
Cogentin (benztropine), 89
cognition, 74, 168
cognitive-behavioral therapy (CBT), 106–9, 121, 191–93
cognitive dysfunction, 26–27, 191–93
cognitive remediation, 26, 111–12, 191–93
cognitive tests, 26, 75–76, 191–93
collateral information, 74–75, 191–93
command hallucinations, 29, 191–93
communication, 134, 143, 167–71, 176*t*, 179–80
community outreach, 65
comorbidity. *See* co-occurring disorder
compulsory treatment. *See* involuntary inpatient treatment
computerized axial tomography (CAT) scan, 77, 191–93
computerized tomography (CT) scan, 77, 191–93
concentration, poor, 26–27, 201–5
confidentiality rules, 78
conventional antipsychotics, 88–91, 89*t*, 191–93
co-occurring disorder, 114, 191–93
coordinated specialty care programs, 59, 61–63, 62*f*, 191–93
coping, 157, 164–67, 191–93
crazy, 6
CT (computerized tomography) scan, 77, 191–93
Cushing's disease, 37–38

day/night reversal, 130, 193–95
day treatment programs, 114–15, 193–95
Decadron (dexamethasone), 39

delirium, 6, 46, 193–95
Deltasone (prednisone), 39
delusional disorder, 44, 193–95
delusion of control, 21, 193–95
delusions, 20–21
    defined, 193–95
    as positive symptom, 4
    responding to, 177–78, 178*f*
dementia, 6, 46–47, 193–95
depression. *See* major depression
derailment. *See* loosening of associations
deterioration in role functioning, 132, 193–95
developing psychosis, 7
dexamethasone (Decadron), 39
diagnoses of psychotic disorders, 18, 35–48, 40*t*
    causes of symptoms, 36–41
        medical causes, 36–38
        psychiatric causes, 39–41
        substances, 38–39
    defined, 193–95
    from evaluation process, 77–78
    other psychiatric disorders causing psychosis, 45–47
    overview, 35–36, 47–48
    primary, 41
        brief psychotic disorder, 41
        delusional disorder, 44
        other specified schizophrenia spectrum and other psychotic disorder, 44
        schizoaffective disorder, 43
        schizophrenia, 42–43
        schizophreniform disorder, 41–42
        unspecified schizophrenia spectrum and other psychotic disorder, 44
Diagnostic and Statistical Manual of Mental Disorders (DSM), 40–41, 193–95
diathesis–stress model, 12, 56*f*, 56, 193–95
diet, 143–45
differential diagnosis, 35–36, 193–95
diphenhydramine (Benadryl), 89
disability, 7, 156–57
disorders, psychotic, 11
disorganization, 23–25, 168, 193–95
disorganized behavior, 25, 193–95
disorientation, 46, 193–95
dissociative identity disorder, 5–6
dopamine, 52–53, 85, 193–95
drive, low, 23, 132–33, 198–99

drug-induced psychosis, 8, 38f, 38–39,
        76, 193–95
DSM (*Diagnostic and Statistical Manual of
        Mental Disorders*), 40–41, 193–95
dual diagnosis. *See* co-occurring disorder
dysphoria, 130, 193–95

Early Assessment and Support Alliance
        (EASA), 62–63
Early Diagnosis and Preventive Treatment
        (EDAPT) program, 62–63
early intervention services, 59, 195
Early Psychosis Prevention and Intervention
        Centre (EPPIC), 60
early warning signs, 129–38
    common, 130–33
    defined, 195
    importance of detecting, 129–30
    overview, 136–38
    recognizing, 174
    relapse prevention, 133–36, 134f
    worksheet, 137
EASA (Early Assessment and Support
        Alliance), 62–63
EDAPT (Early Diagnosis and Preventive
        Treatment) program, 62–63
electroencephalogram (EEG), 37, 76, 195
emergency help, 136, 185–86
emotional withdrawal, 22, 195
encephalopathy, 76
endocrine disorders, 37–38
energy, low, 23, 132–33, 198–99
engagement. *See* sticking with treatment
epilepsy, 37
EPPIC (Early Psychosis Prevention and
        Intervention Centre), 60
EPS (extrapyramidal side effects), 89, 90t, 195
evaluation process, 69–81
    cognitive tests, 75–76
    collateral information, 74–75
    electroencephalogram (EEG), 76
    inpatient versus outpatient
        evaluation, 78–79
    interviews, 70–74
    lab tests, 76
    making diagnosis from, 77–78
    mobile crisis teams, 79–80
    neuroimaging, 76–77
    overview, 80–81
    physical exam, 75

exercise, 143–45
experiences, 7–8
extrapyramidal side effects (EPS), 89, 90t, 195

family and friends
    communication, importance of, 167–71
    coping, 164–66
    early stages of psychosis and, 162
    interventions, 110–11, 196
    psychoeducation, 110–11, 163, 196
    reducing stress, 163
    support for, 124
    support from, 123–24, 145–46
    as supportive environment, 161–72
    therapy, 111, 196
    tips for, 124
fasting glucose and lipids, 93, 196
FDA (Food and Drug Administration),
        92, 144
FIRST Coordinated Specialty Care, 62–63
first-episode psychosis, 5b, 15
    in adolescence, 12
    defined, 5, 196
first-generation antipsychotics. *See*
        conventional antipsychotics
flat affect, 17–18, 22, 196
fluphenazine (Prolixin) decanoate, 95
follow-up appointments, 120
Food and Drug Administration (FDA),
        92, 144
formal thought disorder. *See* disorganization
functional magnetic resonance imaging
        (fMRI), 77

generic name, 83, 196–97
genes, 10, 12, 50–51, 196–97.
        See also risk genes
glucose, 93, 196
glutamate, 52–53, 196–97
grandiose delusion, 20, 196–97
grandiosity, 45–46
grooming, poor attention to, 23, 201–5
group therapy, 109–10, 196–97

Haldol (haloperidol) decanoate, 95
hallucinations, 20. *See also* brief, intermittent
        hallucinations
    defined, 197
    as positive symptom, 4
    responding to, 177–78, 178f

haloperidol (Haldol) decanoate, 95
healthy lifestyle, 139–47, 166–67
    avoiding drugs, 139–43
    change process, 143f
    diet, 143–45
    exercise, 143–45
    overview, 146–47
    sleeping well, 145
    social support, 145–46
heritable, 50–51, 197
histamine, 86, 197
history, gathering, 71
HIV/AIDS, 37–38, 39
hospitalization, 123
hostility, 27, 186–87, 197
hotlines, 79
Huntington's disease, 46–47
hydroxyzine (Atarax, Vistaril), 89
hygiene, poor attention to, 23, 201–5
hypersomnia, 130, 197

ICD (International Classification of
    Diseases), 40–41, 197–98
ideas of reference, 21–22, 131, 197–98
IEP (Individualized Education Plan),
    158, 197–98
imaging studies. See neuroimaging
impaired information processing, 27, 197–98
impaired insight, 25, 197–98
impulse control, 74
inappropriate affect, 28
Individualized Education Plan (IEP),
    158, 197–98
Individual Placement and Support (IPS),
    155–57, 197–98
inpatient evaluation, 70, 78–79
insanity, 6
insight, 74
insomnia, 130, 197–98
integrated treatment programs, 114,
    197–98
intermittent hallucinations. See brief,
    intermittent hallucinations
International Classification of Diseases
    (ICD), 40–41, 197–98
interviews, 70–74
involuntary community treatment. See
    outpatient commitment
involuntary inpatient treatment, 78–79, 123,
    136, 182, 197–98

IPS (Individual Placement and Support),
    155–57, 197–98
irritability, 130

judgment, 74

kidney disease, 37–38

labile affect, 28
lab tests, 76
late-onset schizophrenia, 42–43
life events, 162, 198–99
lipids, 93, 196
liver diseases, 37–38
loosening of associations, 24, 198–99
low-dose medication management, 95
lumbar puncture, 76, 198–99
lunacy, 6
lupus, 37–38

magnetic resonance imaging (MRI), 77,
    199–200
major depression, 43, 45, 108, 199–200
mania, 28, 43, 45–46, 199–200
manic-depressive illness, 10
marijuana, 39, 54, 123
medical causes of psychosis. See psychosis
    related to medical problem
medical record, 71–72
medical steroids, 39
medication induced psychotic disorder.
    See substance/medication induced
    psychotic disorder
medicines. See antipsychotics
memory, poor, 27, 201–5
Mental Health America (MHA), 124, 146, 172
Mental Health First Aid Australia, 173
mental health first aid for psychosis, 173–88
    approaching someone with
        psychosis, 174–75
    being supportive, 176
    communication, 179–80
    hostile behavior, 186–87
    for postnatal psychosis, 183
    professional help, 180–82
        denying, 181–82
        encouraging, 180–81
        supporting, 181
    purpose of, 173
    recognizing psychosis, 174

responding to
    delusions and hallucinations, 177–78
    paranoia, 178–79
self-help strategies, 182–83
severe psychotic state, 183–86
substance use and, 183
suicide risk, 187
talking with someone with psychosis, 175
treating with dignity and respect, 177
Mental Health First Aid program, 173
mental illness, 3–4, 199–200
mental status exam, 72f, 72–74, 199–200
metabolic disorders, 37–38
metabolic side effects, 93, 199–200
methylphenidate (Ritalin), 39
MHA (Mental Health America), 124,
    146, 172
misconceptions and myths about
    psychosis, 5–7
mobile crisis teams, 79–80, 199–200
mood, 73
    changes in, 130
    schizoaffective disorder, 43
    symptom of psychosis, 28
mood stabilizers, 45–46, 96, 199–200
motivation, low, 23, 132–33, 198–99
motivational enhancement therapy, 140–41,
    199–200
motivational interviewing. See motivational
    enhancement therapy
MRI (magnetic resonance imaging), 77,
    199–200
multi-family groups, 199–200
multiple personality disorder, 5–6
myths and misconceptions about
    psychosis, 5–7

Narcotics Anonymous (NA), 142
National Academy of Sleep Medicine, 145
National Alliance on Mental Illness (NAMI),
    124, 146, 172
National Institute of Mental Health
    (NIMH), 60
negative symptoms, 4, 22–23, 34
    with cognitive dysfunction, 26
    defined, 200–1
    interfering with communication, 168
neurocognitive tests. See cognitive tests
neurodevelopmental model, 12, 200–1
neuroimaging, 76–77, 200–1

neuroleptics. See conventional antipsychotics
neurons, 52, 200–1
neuropsychological tests. See cognitive tests
neurotransmitters, 52, 200–1
nicotine replacement therapy, 140–41,
    141t, 200–1
NIMH (National Institute of Mental
    Health), 60
N-methyl-D-aspartate (NMDA) receptor
    autoimmune encephalitis, 37–38
non-bizarre delusions, 21
norepinephrine, 86, 200–1
normal experiences, 7–8

olanzapine (Zyprexa), 93
ongoing stressors, 162, 201
online resources
    Mental Health First Aid program, 173,
        183, 187
    specialty care programs, 67
OnTrackNY program, 62–63
open dialogue, 111, 201
other specified schizophrenia spectrum and
        other psychotic disorder, 44, 201
outpatient commitment, 70, 79, 201
outpatient evaluation, 78–79
overvalued ideas, 131, 201

paliperidone, 95
paranoia. See suspiciousness
paranoid delusion, 20, 201–5
Parkinson's disease, 39, 46–47
partial hospitalization programs,
        114–15, 201–5
peer specialists, 59b, 59, 153, 201–5
peer support, 153, 201–5
perceptual abnormality, 132, 201–5
PET (positron emission tomography)
        scan, 77
physical exam, 75
planning, difficulties with, 27, 193–95
positive symptoms, 4, 13–14, 20–22, 34
    clozapine (Clozaril) and, 93–94
    defined, 201–5
    delusions, 20–21
    hallucinations, 20
    ideas of reference, 21–22
    interfering with communication,
        167–68
    suspiciousness/paranoia, 21

positron emission tomography (PET)
    scan, 77
postpartum psychosis, 45, 183, 201–5
poverty of content of speech, 24, 201–5
prednisone (Deltasone), 39
pregnancy, 52f
primary psychotic disorders, 18, 41, 49–56
  brief psychotic disorder, 41
  defined, 201–5
  delusional disorder, 44
  external risk factors, 50–51, 51f
    abnormalities in brain development,
      52–53, 54–55
    during childhood and
      adolescence, 53–54
    genes, 50–51
  other specified schizophrenia spectrum
      and other psychotic disorder, 44
  schizoaffective disorder, 43
  schizophrenia, 42–43
  schizophreniform disorder, 41–42
  unspecified schizophrenia spectrum and
      other psychotic disorder, 44
prodromal phase, 12–13, 66, 201–5
prodromal symptoms, 4, 18, 29–30, 34, 201–5
professional help, 180–82
  denying, 181–82
  encouraging, 180–81
  supporting, 181
prolactin, 89–90, 201–5
Prolixin (fluphenazine) decanoate, 95
psychiatric advance directive, 184–85, 201–5
psychiatric causes of psychosis, 39–41
psychiatrists, 35b, 70–71, 134, 201–5
psychoeducation, 63b, 63, 164, 201–5
psychoeducational groups, 109, 201–5
psychologists, 70–71, 201–5
psychopathy, 6
psychosis, 3–15
  defined, 3–5, 201–5
  developing, 7
  diagnoses, 35–48
  disorders, 45–47
  key points, 15
  myths and misconceptions about, 5–7
  possible causes of, 12
  psychosis continuum, 7–11
  recognizing, 174
  schizophrenia, 11
  symptoms, 17–34, 19t

catatonia, 27–28
causes of, 36–41
cognitive dysfunction, 26–27
disorganization, 23–25
hostility, 27
impaired insight, 25
mood and anxiety, 28
negative, 22–23
overview, 17–18, 30, 34
positive, 20–22
prodromal, 29–30
suicidal thoughts, 29
symptoms checklist worksheet, 31–33
treatment and recovery, 12–14
psychosis continuum, 7–11, 9f, 201–5
psychosis-prone, 10, 201–5
psychosis related to medical problem, 36–38,
    37f, 201–5
psychosocial development, 103–4, 201–5
psychosocial rehabilitation, 104, 201–5
psychosocial treatments, 64b, 64–65,
    103–18, 107t
assertive community treatment
    (ACT), 115
cognitive-behavioral therapy
    (CBT), 106–9
cognitive remediation, 111–12
day treatment programs, 114–15
defined, 201–5
family interventions, 110–11
group therapy, 109–10
overview, 116–18
partial hospitalization programs, 114–15
psychosocial development, 103–4
purpose of, 104–5
social skills training, 113
starting, 105–6
substance use treatment programs, 114
supported employment and
    education, 112–13
supportive housing, 115–16
worksheet, 116
psychotic, 201–5
psychotic depression, 45
psychotic disorder, 4, 201–5
psychotic episode, 4, 7, 201–5

RAISE (Recovery After an Initial
    Schizophrenia Episode), 60–61
receptors, 85, 205–6

recovery, 12–14, 149–54
  characteristics of, 152
  defined, 205–6
  model, 149–50
  overview, 153–54
  peer support, 153
  principles of, 150f, 150–52
Recovery After an Initial Schizophrenia
      Episode (RAISE), 60–61
recovery model, 42, 205–6
recovery phase, 12–13, 205–6
referrals, 105, 205–6
relapse, 123. See also sticking with treatment
  defined, 205–6
  prevention, 129, 133–36, 134f, 205–6
  prodromal symptoms and, 29–30
relaxation, 166
religious delusion, 20, 205–6
remission, 98, 149, 205–6
risk factors, 50–51
  abnormalities in brain development,
      52–53, 54–55
  during childhood and adolescence, 53–54
  defined, 49, 205–6
risk genes, 51, 205–6
risperidone (Risperdal), 89–90, 95
Ritalin (methylphenidate), 39

sadness, 130
schizoaffective disorder, 43, 206–10
schizoaffective disorder-bipolar type,
      43, 206–10
schizoaffective disorder-depressive type,
      43, 206–10
schizophrenia, 11, 42–43, 49–56
  age of onset, 7
  defined, 206–10
  external risk factors, 50–51
    abnormalities in brain development,
      52–53, 54–55
    during childhood and
      adolescence, 53–54
  genes, 50–51
schizophreniform disorder, 41–42, 206–10
schizotypal personality disorder, 10,
      46, 206–10
schizotypal personality features, 10, 206–10
school. See supported education and
      employment
secondary negative symptoms, 88–89

second-generation antipsychotics. See
      atypical antipsychotics
seizure disorder, 37
self-harm, 4
self-help strategies, 182–83
serotonin, 86, 91, 206–10
severe psychotic state, 183–86
severity, 8, 206–10
shared decision-making, 61–62,
      119–20, 206–10
side effects, 87t
  of antipsychotics, 86–87
  defined, 206–10
signs, 17–18, 206–10
single photon emission computed
      tomography (SPECT) scan, 77
sleep, 145
  disturbance, 130
  medicines, 96, 206–10
slow movements, 23, 206–10
smoking cessation, 140–41
  defined, 206–10
  medicines for, 140–41, 206–10
social isolation, 23, 206–10
social skills, 64–65, 113, 206–10
social skills training, 113, 206–10
social withdrawal, 132, 206–10
sociopathy, 6
somatic delusion, 21, 206–10
Specialized Treatment Early in Psychosis
      (STEP) program, 62–63
specialty care programs, 59–67
  case management, 63
  community outreach, 65
  coordinated specialty care
      programs, 61–63
  growth of, 60–61
  medicines, 64
  peer specialists, 153
  prodromal phase treatment, 66
  psychoeducation, 63
  psychosocial treatments, 64–65
  services provided, 61b, 61
SPECT (single photon emission computed
      tomography) scan, 77
speech, 23, 73, 206–10
spinal tap. See lumbar puncture
spirituality, 166
STEP (Specialized Treatment Early in
      Psychosis) program, 62–63

steroids, medical, 39
sticking with treatment, 119–25
    difficulties with, 122
    duration of treatment, 122
    family and friends, 123–24
    follow-up appointments, 120
    hospitalization, 123
    importance of, 123
    overview, 125
    practicing new skills, 121
    shared decision-making, 119–20
    taking medicine as prescribed,
        120–21
stigma, 153, 206–10
stress
    communication, importance of, 167–71
    coping, 164–67
    defined, 162, 206–10
    early stages of psychosis and, 162
    overview, 171–72
    reducing, 135
      in family, 163
      people with psychosis, 164
stressful life events, 53–54, 123, 206–10
stress-induced psychosis, 8, 206–10
stressors, 162, 206–10
strokes, 46–47
substance/medication induced psychotic
        disorder, 8, 38–39
substance use, 4, 183
    during adolescence, 54
    avoiding, 139–43
    minimizing, 135
    treatment programs, 114
substance use disorder, 139–40, 206–10
suicidal thoughts, 29, 187, 206–10
supported education and employment,
        112–13, 155–60
    defined, 206–10
    disclosure of mental illness, 159
    importance of, 155–56
    overview, 159–60
    supports for going back to, 156–58
supportive housing, 115–16, 206–10
supportive psychotherapy, 109, 206–10
suspiciousness, 21, 131, 178–79, 206–10
symptoms of psychosis, 17–34. *See also* early
        warning signs
    catatonia, 27–28
    causes of, 36–41
      medical causes, 36–38

      psychiatric causes, 39–41
      substances, 38–39
    cognitive dysfunction, 26–27
    defined, 206–10
    disorganization, 23–25
    hostility, 27
    impaired insight, 25
    mood and anxiety, 28
    negative, 22–23
    overview, 17–18, 30, 34
    positive, 20–22
      delusions, 20–21
      hallucinations, 20
      ideas of reference, 21–22
      suspiciousness/paranoia, 21
    prodromal, 29–30
    suicidal thoughts, 29
    symptoms checklist worksheet, 31–33
syndrome of psychosis. *See* psychotic
        episode
syndromes, 17, 206–10

tangentiality, 24, 210
tardive dyskinesia (TD), 90–91, 210
temporal lobe epilepsy, 37–38, 76
tension, 130
therapy groups, 110, 210
thinking
    difficulties with abstract, 26, 193–95
    slow or empty, 23, 206–10
thought blocking, 24, 131, 210
thought content, 73–74
thought disorder. *See* disorganization
thought process, 73
tobacco, 139
trade name, 83, 210
treatment, 12–14
treatment-resistant psychosis, 94, 210
trihexyphenidyl (Artane), 89
12-step program, 114, 189
typical antipsychotics. *See* conventional
      antipsychotics

unawareness of illness. *See* impaired insight
unspecified schizophrenia spectrum
      and other psychotic
      disorder, 44, 210–11
USDA MyPlate program, 144

varenicline (Chantix), 140–41
violence, 6–7

Vistaril (hydroxyzine), 89
vocational rehabilitation, 112–13
voluntary inpatient treatment, 78–79, 79*b*,
    123, 211

weight gain, 93, 211
Wellbutrin (bupropion), 140–41
work. *See* supported education and
    employment

working diagnosis, 35–36, 36*b*, 211
worksheets
    early warning signs, 137
    medicines prescribed, 100
    psychosocial treatments, 116
    symptoms checklist, 31–33

Zyban (bupropion), 140–41
Zyprexa (olanzapine), 93